Anorexia: A Son's Battle, A Mother's War

Debbie Roche

ISBN-13: 978-1522761006:
ISBN-10: 1522761004

DEDICATION

To my beloved David.

For his limitless patience, understanding and wit which kept me going through the low, desperate and pressured times...and the writing of this book!

CONTENTS

ACKNOWLEDGEMENTS

First of all, I wish to acknowledge the mighty strength and extraordinary resolve of all mums, dads and carers currently caring for a child living with an eating disorder - you are all amazing!

I also wish to personally thank Sam Thomas of Men Get Eating Disorders Too and Fran Marriott for their invaluable friendship, knowledge and expertise. Furthermore, I wish to thank Debra Schlesinger and the mothers of Mothers Against Eating Disorders for providing priceless online sisterly support.

Finally, I wish to thank GeorgeSpade@123rf.com for the amazing cover image that is so befitting of the personal battles contained within the book.

PREFACE

When my teenage son was diagnosed with anorexia nervosa, I was totally unprepared for the path of devastation that lay ahead. I had no idea of the anguish, pain and tears that the tortuous eating disorder had in store for us. I feel that had I been better aware of the toxic traits of anorexia then maybe, just maybe, our family might have been saved from the truly destructive ordeals that the condition imposed upon us. As Mum, I endured some of the most agonising moments of my life. As if grief from losing my son's teenage years wasn't enough, the guilt I experienced from not recognising such a vehement enemy in the home was excruciating.

My physical being became hostage to the emotional and psychological torture constantly exerted by the eating disorder.

Debbie Roche

Nonetheless, I was resolute in my determination to fight the eating disorder. Accordingly, I commenced my own reconnaissance mission. Slowly I got to know the enemy and began to devise a battle strategy, one which would take years to deliver. This book is part of my arsenal of war.

Through endless unconditional love and sheer determination, the adversity that the challenges of the eating disorder posed has been surpassed. I have weathered the intensity and perplexity of my son's condition. I feel that I am now in a position to expose the virulent features and characteristics of not only anorexia but other eating disorders.

This book is a tapestry of my experiences, perceptions and acquired knowledge throughout the devastating times when anorexia nervosa, a potential killer, infiltrated my home. The chapters of this book, which hopefully prove to be interesting and informative reading, are the consequences of my determination to see the eating disorder forced out of our lives.

Furthermore, this book is also intended to be a useful source of ammunition for other families who may find themselves taunted and

2

defiled by an eating disorder in the home. By raising awareness of the evil and dangers that eating disorders pose to our children and other loved ones, parents and carers will be equipped to effectively fight eating disorders - the scourge of the 21st century.

1. AS IT WAS IN THE BEGINNING

"I found myself faced with the most frightening, devastating and incomprehensible situation that any parent would quake at. I was witnessing my gorgeous son slowly kill himself."

Ollie, my youngest child of three, was a particularly happy and content child - always smiling and cracking jokes of his own brand of childlike humour. I am sure you know the jokes I mean. The ones that children alone find hilarious but adults laugh uncontrollably at because the logic behind the joke is so…well, funny!

Like so many youngsters, my son was captivated by the ever popular Japanese anime series, Pokémon, a story of a young boy and his amazing fun-filled journeys around the world whilst fulfilling his passion for catching and training magnificent insects and other forms of life. He used to hold dear a plush figure of Charmander, one of the cartoon's little fire breathing creatures. It went everywhere with him.

And he used to love the Friday fight nights. To be honest these particular nights were the highlight of my week. I recall all of the family eagerly hovering around the lounge, with lap trays in hand, embellished with a plate of tasty Chinese takeaway and a glass of fizz, seeking out our preferred seats in front of the television in order to get ringside view of the amazing Stone Cold Steve Austin, The Rock, Lita and The Hardy Boys.

But there were two sides to Ollie - the bright, happy little boy and his alter-ego, the unwell, sad little boy. Ollie often complained of general un-wellness: stomach pains, leg pains, shoulder pains. He was always acquiring injuries whilst participating in school sports, tag rugby or whatever other sport he was playing.

To be perfectly honest he actually tallied up quite a number of GP appointments in his early years - but neither did his early teens escape the tribulations of physical ailments. Indeed, the general un-wellness continued throughout his early teens and along with the onset of 'dark episodes' in his mind, so did the GP appointments.

One day there must have been some sort of 'Eureka' moment for Ollie's GP. For some reason, whether it was a flash of inspiration or the determination to fight the ritual of surgery attendances, the doctor referred Ollie for a series of face-to-face counselling sessions. The counselling sessions were not to be provided by the in-house team, but by a local organisation which dealt solely with young people and their issues.

Of course, the intention of these sessions was to assist him in not only trying to recognise some of the frustrations he was experiencing, but also to help him sift through those frustrations before they became major life difficulties. However, the therapy didn't even scratch the surface. Ollie's dark patch continued to darken; it became deeper and wider by each passing day and everyone was blind to this - including me!

Over the following weeks Ollie's ailments became more severe and destructive. His stamina waned and strength dissipated. It became evident that Ollie was not eating enough to manage his daily routines - another visit to the GP was required. The GP prescribed a course of thick, highly nutritious, supplement drinks. Available in a variety of flavours, Ollie's taste buds would certainly benefit, but would Ollie?

Initially, Ollie appeared keen to see the course of treatment through. I was relieved at the thought that whatever was medically wrong was now being addressed. To my dismay, my relief was soon obliterated. My endeavours to persuade and encourage him to stay focused on completing the flavoursome treatment failed.

After a couple of days he began to vehemently protest. He would make himself retch at the very thought of putting one of the drinks to his lips. Unfortunately, his protestations didn't remain with the supplement drinks - he began to refuse all manner of foods, and even began to dislike drinking water. I found myself faced with the most frightening, devastating and incomprehensible situation that any parent would quake at. I was witnessing my gorgeous son slowly kill himself. I was powerless to save him from whatever malevolent force was gripping him.

Fortunately, the GP had recognised the severity of my son's condition and suitably sent in the cavalry, by way of a psychiatrist and the Child and Adolescent Mental Health Services (CAMHS), a multidisciplinary service providing specialist mental health services to children and young people, including those with severe, complex and persistent mental health needs.

Despite expecting the visit, I admit to being rather anxious about the psychiatrist's impending appearance at my door. I must have tread a weary track on the hallway carpet that day as I waited for the doorbell to ring!

Ding, dong. As the ringing doorbell announced the visitor's arrival, Ollie and I glanced fleetingly at each other. I noticed that his eyes were dark and wide with fear and dread - no doubt that he noticed that of me. Nonetheless, with clammy hands, I clumsily opened the door.

There stood the psychiatrist, nothing at all as I expected. I smiled hesitantly, and she in return. In trepidation, I welcomed her into our little sanctuary. The countdown to diagnosis had commenced.

I was first to be interviewed which, in all honesty, was an opportunity I actually welcomed. I constantly repeated to myself, "She's here to make things better for Ollie. She's here to make things better." But the words didn't alter the fact that I was churning inside. A diagnosis would set us on the path to recovery. We would have access to appropriate treatment and professionals.

The psychiatrist positioned herself on the chair opposite me. Without delay, she deftly placed a large black leather notebook on her lap. From her oversized brown bag she pulled out a silver coloured roller ball pen and slowly depressed the top. Click. The interview thus began.

I felt extremely uncomfortable with the questions she asked - quite personal and intrusive. Delving into my marriage, divorce, relationship with my parents and mental health history. I felt as if I was the suspect of a heinous crime rather than trying to help with my son's situation.

Despite being aware that I could decline to answer any question she posed, the answers just fell from my mouth, like a case of verbal diarrhoea. Whether it was my nervousness, the psychiatrist's complete calm and modulation or even my sub-conscious thought that every answer would help Ollie's case I can't say, but I was thankful when it was over.

After an hour or so, it was Ollie's turn to grace the makeshift interrogation room and, for one fleeting moment as we quickly shifted to our respective rooms, our eyes met. Fear was still firmly entrenched in Ollie's dark eyes. I wanted to crumple and cry.

Within what appeared to be no time at all, the psychiatrist called me back into the room. I felt sick - so painfully nauseous. My head was heavy, frantically dancing with the unknown. I parked myself next to Ollie on the sofa and awaited the deliberations of the psychiatrist.

As I had suspected, the news wasn't good. Her softly spoken voice delivered a haunting diagnosis of anorexia nervosa. My entire world shattered into a million pieces. My head began to viciously pound as my heart swiftly sank deep down into the pit of my stomach.

As guilt permeated my very being, I began to panic at my lack of preparedness for such news and dread at the uncertainty for the future. Naturally I was wholly devastated at the diagnosis. Astonishingly however, I also had a conflicting feeling of relief.

After months and months of visits to the GP for various complaints, treatment for this, that and the other, my son's condition had finally been diagnosed and he would finally begin to receive the treatment he desperately needed.

I cannot begin to explain just how indigestible it was to hear that my teenage son had developed such an unimaginable condition, particularly one that is normally associated with adolescent girls and their delusions of fame and super-stardom. Being a parent is a challenge in itself, but being the parent of a child with an eating disorder is a profoundly daunting role.

As a former health and social care lecturer, I thought I was fairly well-informed about eating disorders - but my son's diagnosis clearly illustrated that I wasn't and this disappointed me terribly. I didn't see the signs of the lurking, contemptuous eating disorder and this made me feel guilty and utterly ashamed.

My ignorance and lack of knowledge had helped the eating disorder firmly root itself into my son's being and it wasn't going to be an easy task to remove it, particularly as I wasn't appropriately equipped with the weapons to fight it. With the best weapon in the world being knowledge, I went on a personal mission to learn everything I possibly could about anorexia.

Following the psychiatrist's diagnosis, Ollie was referred to the CAMHS Outreach Service which aims to provide support to children and young people within their own homes and communities.

The two mental health professionals assigned to Ollie's case could not have been more suitably matched. Both appeared to have an excellent understanding of his condition - of its manipulative, cruel, devious and dangerous nature. But more importantly, they appeared approachable, friendly, pleasant and good humoured - personal qualities which allowed for an almost instantaneous rapport on which he could build a strong, trusting and respectful relationship. As it happens this relationship proved to be especially invaluable when Ollie was at one of his most vulnerable and defenceless moments.

2. MALEVOLENCE LAYING IN WAIT

"...his torso, sunken and sallow, resembled the carcass of a well-devoured Sunday

lunch chicken. His skin, tissue-paper thin and webbed with fine broken veins,

covered his bony ribcage."

The previously hidden loathsome condition began to show its true, utter contempt for Ollie. In one fell swoop, the many months of weight loss, spates of dizziness, lethargy and malaise, and other multitude of ailments finally presented themselves. His physical being, seemingly exempt of energy, could no longer handle the fight - he coiled himself up on the sofa. It was abundantly clear that something drastic needed to be done for him.

Fortunately, I managed to obtain an emergency GP appointment. Even before the doctor had concluded the physical examination, she mooted her thoughts about Ollie needing to go to hospital for a more thorough, in-depth physical examination. Within no time we were at Derriford Hospital. After a series of routine tests, which included a complete blood count and electrolyte and protein checks, Ollie was deemed sufficiently stable to return home.

A few days later an intensive intervention package comprising of daily home visits by the CAMHS Outreach Team, weekly blood tests, plus twice-weekly physical monitoring by the GP, was established. To say I was relieved at this point is an understatement. However, things did not progress as hoped.

One week later, on 5th November, as a consequence of worsening physical statistics, reports of dizziness, lethargy and weakness, courtesy of an ambulance, Ollie was rushed to hospital.

Terrified and panicked, he was duly admitted to the Wildgoose Ward, a ward for young people aged between twelve and sixteen years. The bright lights of the ward did nothing to hide his terror. However, I was determined that nothing would expose my angst - for Ollie's sake. The last thing he needed was an over-anxious, fretting mother at his bedside. So, whilst keeping one eye on Ollie's disposition, I fixed the other on the professionals as they swiftly carried out their duties.

The whole experience felt quite surreal. It all seemed very bizarre. My senses seemed to be in overdrive. For instance, as I sat by Ollie's bed, there was an eerie feel, a strange coldness around my neck. The bed Ollie was resting in appeared too big and out of sync for his slight frame. The hefty stiff-cotton covered pillows shrouded his head which gave the impression of him sinking into a host of white cotton-wool cumulus clouds. My hearing became distorted. I was overwhelmed by the stressful situation.

The medical professionals decided Ollie required an ECG (electrocardiograph) to chart his heart's activity. This procedure required the securing of tiny sound inducers to his chest. Everything seemed to be happening at lightning speed. However, it wasn't until the equipment was rushed to the side of his bed that I began to view the situation in real time. I began to take stock of the severity of the occasion.

Reluctantly, whilst not relishing the examination, Ollie slowly leant forward and awkwardly clasped the bottom of his T-shirt. With eyes full of dread he stole a subtle glance in my direction and whooshed the garment over his head. Smack! My whole body wobbled as it received an almighty overload of repulsion. It was the first time in nearly two years that I had seen Ollie's bare chest, and it's a vision that is going to haunt me forever.

The true extent of the malice that the eating disorder had subjected my son to was abundantly and shockingly apparent. As he sank back on the metal framed bed, his torso, sunken and sallow, resembled the carcass of a well-devoured Sunday lunch chicken. His skin, tissue-paper thin and webbed with fine broken veins, covered his bony ribcage.

I tried so desperately hard not to stare at the sunken vessel that was supposedly my son, but I couldn't avoid it. His emaciated body overwhelmed my very being. I felt ungraciously sick - and full of guilt. Yet again, I began to question my idiotic ignorance of the vicious condition.

I cannot pinpoint when the malevolent anorexia began to develop, but I can provide possible suggestions as to why Ollie acquired it. It is widely mentioned that in order for an eating disorder to occur key factors have to be present - namely predisposing and precipitating factors.[1]

Predisposing factors are factors already pertinent to the individual before the eating disorder develops. In effect they could be called pre-requisites, as without these base factors the eating disorder would not be triggered into existence. Precipitating factors are also known as triggering factors. In essence, eating disorders will develop if the foundations of vulnerability are in place. On reflection, there are a number of likely factors which over time could have contributed to Ollie acquiring anorexia.

His personality. Ollie was a very pleasant, considerate, empathic, sensitive and caring young boy. Great personal qualities which remain with him today. He was intelligent, sensible, pleasant and polite. Willing to help people wherever he could, he always went out of his way to please people. From what I witnessed, he enjoyed being the young knight in shining armour. I never had any cause to worry about him.

Conversely, and on a less positive note, he was rather subservient and compliant to the whims of his siblings. Rightly or wrongly, I perceived his relationship with his brother and sister to be a normal part of the familial hierarchy. As the third child, Ollie was constantly faced with situations where he found himself compromising and negotiating for affection, attention and acknowledgement.

Fortunately, with the benefit of therapy, he has relayed to me how he felt when he was growing up. He felt so side-lined and isolated, as if everything he said wasn't listened to or even heard. In other words, he felt invisible.

Over the years, Ollie developed skills which allowed him to court harmonious relationships with his siblings. He adapted to a life of 'agreeance', which made his relationships with his siblings easier and happier.

On the surface he appeared content with the identity he had carved for himself. He was good-natured; cheerful; creative; a delight to be with - little did I know that this was a camouflage, a façade to cover his innermost feelings of insecurity, poor self-esteem and low self-worth. He was nurturing an identity crisis - a conflict between understanding himself as Ollie, his true personality and his relationships with others.

According to various pieces I have read in relation to personality and eating disorders, Ollie bears traits of a personality style labelled sociotropy. Sociotropy is a combination of an individual's attitudes, beliefs and interactions that steer towards personal satisfaction based on dependency and attention to others.[2&3]

Sociotropic people are concerned with acceptance and approval from others. They avoid confrontation in an attempt to avert abandonment. Regrettably, due to the inherent perplexities of human relationships, this makes them more susceptible to mental ill health, such as depression and high anxiety.

Ollie was also a very conscientious, hard-working young boy - of which his early school reports illustrate - and I would say quite a perfectionist. Indeed, some research suggests perfectionism is a characteristic of an avoidant personality, a characteristic which features highly in people with anorexia.[4]

He would plough himself into school work, art, personal projects and such like - endlessly striving for that ultimate piece of work. He paid avid attention to his appearance, always wanting to be dressed well. On reflection, this attention to model detail started whilst at primary school. I recall how he used to decide what outfit he wanted to wear around the age of five.

As previously mentioned, it is extremely difficult to pinpoint when the anorexia started. Whilst some of the predisposing factors have been identified, I question as to what it was exactly that triggered the eating disorder into existence. I could hasten a few guesses.

Ollie had to cope with many emotional upheavals when he was a small child. His father and I separated when he was five years old. Of course, separation is a very difficult time for everyone. However, for a young child such an experience inflicts emotions such as sense of loss, rejection, anger, guilt and self-blame that are very difficult for them to explain.

Furthermore, the situation could provoke feelings of insecurity which could have an effect on their behaviour. Indeed, during this period there were clear indicators that the situation was upsetting Ollie. Although he couldn't verbally express his feelings, his behavioural changes said so much.

His drawings, once full of colour, became rather distressing pieces of work. Happy characters were replaced with images of people crying.

He also began to wet the bed, something he hadn't done since potty training.

In addition to the distressing situation at home, his early school days were not the happiest of his life. Unfortunately, his left-handedness became a topic of contention. Despite there being substantial studies evidencing advantages of being a left-hander, he was pilloried at primary school for being so.

I recall how one of his first primary school teachers had a quiet word with me because of his apparent motor difficulties. She mentioned the difficulty Ollie experienced in putting his coat on. This in turn assisted in creating moments of unrest with his peers as they lined up to leave the building at the end of the day. I felt so incensed by her comments.

He managed to dress himself at home so what was the problem at school? Naturally he didn't have the urgency that the school teacher probably imposed upon him. I duly reminded the teacher that Ollie was left-handed and sometimes things needed to be demonstrated to him differently. The school teacher did not take into account that the brain of a left-hander works differently. It is known that left-handers respond better to having a mirror image to copy. Handing Ollie his coat the same way as other children and expecting the same result was futile - it simply wasn't going to happen.

But it wasn't only members of staff that attacked his self-confidence. His so-called poor co-ordination and slowness saw him ridiculed by his peers. Even the most simple of tasks in the classroom would create anxiety for him. Whilst his fellow classmates would sail through paper craft sessions, he would struggle with the tasks, particularly as he was not given left-handed scissors to work with. Such experiences could have caused Ollie great emotional pain and subsequently contributed to a cache of precipitating factors for the eating disorder.

To sum up - my youngest son was an insecure, highly sensitive, caring, perfectionist with personal experiences creating deep, emotional pain. He was indeed a vulnerable boy possessing some of the predisposing factors awaiting the precipitating factors to facilitate the onset of anorexia nervosa - a condition laying in wait - to kill.

3. NIGHT BEFORE THE STORM

"I so desperately wanted to be refreshed from the excruciating images of Ollie's wan and deformed body."

I can't remember my first thoughts and emotions on the morning following Ollie's rushed admittance to hospital...but I can remember feeling devastatingly numb. Unsurprisingly, I had had a rather upsettingly sleepless night.

Previously soaked with salty tears of anguish and woe, my now tight-skinned face burned with tiredness and constant disbelief. It was hard to see anything through my bleary eyes, never mind trying to focus on even the simplest of functions such as feeding the cat (which was a very messy activity, getting more food on her and the floor than in the bowl). Even making my morning cup of Earl Grey tea proved a dangerous mission, opening myself to minor scalding mishaps in the process. My fuzzy brain so wanted the events of the night before to be a dream - but they weren't.

Regardless of what I wanted to believe, I knew Ollie was seriously ill and, despite him being in the care of expert healthcare professionals, I knew that he needed me by his side. It was necessary for me to return to the hospital - pronto!

In a meagre attempt to wake myself from my harrowing nightmare, I decided to indulge in one of my occasional mindful moments - taking a long, hot, relaxing shower. With shaking hands pressing the tiled wall for balance, I awkwardly stepped into the white enamelled bath and assumed my usual position under the shower head.

Click. My whole body tingled as the gushing water worked hard to cleanse me of the previous day's mental pains. And, as the rejuvenating water hit my face, I closed my eyes and tried to immerse my thoughts into plans for the future, positive plans for the future. I so desperately wanted to be refreshed from the excruciating images of Ollie's wan and deformed body - but to no avail. The visions remained and so did the mental pain and anguish.

The melancholic four mile return to Derriford Hospital appeared to take hours, for a whole host of reasons. At the time I felt sure that there was a conspiracy to prevent me from getting to my desperate destination. It was as if all of the pedestrians in Plymouth had transcended on the route to the hospital to monopolise every pedestrian crossing! The taxi seemed to stop at every set of traffic lights...not to mention the tailback. My desire for an expeditious drive was irrevocably replaced with the want to just get to see Ollie that morning!

Feeling tired and outright shocking, looking dishevelled and totally ill-prepared for the unknown, I eventually arrived at the hospital. Wearily, I made my way to the ward where Ollie had been admitted.

The walk to his bedside was long, protracted and quite surreal. The corridors seemed to stretch for miles and miles - they were never-ending! Each somnolent step I took was like being put through my paces on a treadmill - constantly moving but getting nowhere. Anxious and apprehensive, I arrived at my son's bedside at what appeared to be a rather desperate time. Ollie looked petrified. His sunken eyes were wide with fear and, whatever negligible colour he had had the day before had seriously drained from him. I was horrified to see him in such a state. After all, he was in hospital and I would expect an improved not reduced condition.

Despite his obvious physical and mental turmoil, Ollie in a composed yet surprisingly animated manner, relayed particular substantial events of the morning to me. It materialised that the doctor, in her so-called wisdom, had decided to give Ollie a lesson on the impact and serious effects that anorexia has on the body's muscles - especially the heart.

Anorexia presents numerous consequences for the physical health of the sufferer. I would like to add here that whilst I do not like the term sufferer, individuals living with an eating disorder do experience degrees of suffering, hence my reason for using such a negative word. Some of the consequences are visible to the eye, i.e. lanugo (soft, fine downy hair) and others are invisible, such as osteoporosis; damage to the internal organs; lowered potassium levels.

Potassium is an extremely important mineral for the body for muscles require potassium to be able to contract. The heart muscle however, also needs potassium to be able to beat properly as well as regulate the blood pressure. Because Ollie was experiencing an advanced stage of anorexia, his heart was losing muscle mass. In effect, his body was eating itself.

There was no wonder at all that my son was feeling terrified. As for me, I was absolutely livid. I could not, and still cannot, comprehend the logic and total lack of sensitivity of that professional. Indeed, one of the first things I read about talking to your child with an eating disorder was not to make them feel guilty or try to blackmail them about their condition. I was gobsmacked!

I suppose like any caring and protective parent, my initial reaction was to seek out the doctor and vent my spleen for upsetting my ill son - something I know I would have regretted later. But Ollie, the eternal pacifist, begged me not to say or do anything - he just wanted to get out of the hospital as quickly as possible, by any means possible.

However, it wasn't only Ollie that was looking in a worse state than when I left him the day before - his CAMHS support staff were looking equally irritated, frustrated and angry. It transpired that not ten minutes before I had arrived at the hospital, the decision to intubate Ollie with a nasogastric tube (NGT) had been the topic of a heated, behind the curtain, discussion.

For the benefit of those not familiar with the term - a nasogastric tube is a small, soft plastic tube which is inserted through the nasal canal, past the pharynx and down the oesophagus (gullet/food pipe) into the stomach. The purpose of this rather uncommon procedure is to deliver comprehensive and appropriate feeding formulae directly into the stomach.

Indeed, there are many stories of people living with the evils of anorexia nervosa that have been at the receiving end of such treatment. Parents have blogged about how demeaning and inhuman the life-saving procedure felt to them. Hand on heart, I know I would have been absolutely devastated had he been subjected to the heinous nasogastric tube.

Fortunately for Ollie and me, the attending CAMHS team were fervently opposed to such a procedure and they made their feelings vigorously known to the presiding doctor. In their wisdom they offered, in my opinion, an equitable alternative to the proffered course of action - inpatient stay at the nearby young person's psychiatric hospital.

Although undeniably very shocked at the prospect of Ollie's admittance to such an establishment, I understood that it was not uncommon for young people suffering with the extreme late-stages of an eating disorder to experience a period as an inpatient which in many cases, provided a valuable route to recovery.

Of course, I appreciate that recovery from an eating disorder for one person is not the same for someone else. The relapses and setbacks Ollie would face whilst on the path to recovery would be time consuming and depressingly difficult to manage. The young person's unit would provide the appropriate professional support necessary to assist Ollie on his journey to recovery.

The thought of my son missing out on all of his teenage years was heartbreaking. If Ollie stood any chance of regaining his life then this proposal was definitely the lifeline we both needed.

4. INPATIENT CHARM

"His heart had suffered greatly from the self-imposed starvation that the eating disorder had inflicted, therefore rest and no exertion were paramount to Ollie's care in the unit."

I consider myself one of the more fortunate parents in terms of inpatient stay. I lived in close proximity to the young person's unit - only a mile away from home - which allowed not only frequent and quick access to Ollie, but also enabled perpetual attendance at the family therapy sessions.

Through conversations I have had, I know that some parents were not as fortunate. One young patient's mother had a round trip of one hundred and forty miles. With other caring responsibilities at home this prevented her from frequently seeing her unwell loved one.

Ollie's first few days as an inpatient were particularly daunting for him. His poor physical condition, blood pressure, frailty, weakened heart and other health complications associated with anorexia nervosa, restricted his mobility so much that he was consigned to a manually-operated wheelchair. Furthermore, as he did not have the strength to operate the chair himself, he had to be pushed around the unit by a member of staff.

This reliance upon a member of staff for mobility was extremely difficult for him to bear - especially as it included visits to the toilet. Not only did he feel embarrassed at being escorted to the toilet, he felt uncomfortable trying to 'function' whilst the staff member waited for him outside. Ollie had no personal private time. He had lost his freedom of movement, and also his dignity.

I accept that, frustrating though it was for Ollie, restricting his mobility was an important feature for his care and promotion of recovery. His heart had suffered greatly from the self-imposed starvation that the eating disorder had inflicted, therefore rest and no exertion were paramount to Ollie's care in the unit. However, I do not accept that the varying degrees of care provided at the unit were beneficial features of his care and recovery. In my opinion, there was a distinct divide between the services provided.

On one hand, Ollie had access to some of the most exceptional psychotherapy and family therapy, delivered by seemingly specialised and knowledgeable professionals. Whereas on the other hand, many of the general day-to-day staff appeared to lack not only the knowledge and understanding of anorexia nervosa, but also the skills base to manage patients with the condition.

According to relayed experiences, there appeared to be an unforgivable, acute lack of verbal communication skills with regard to anorexic patients - an issue I enthusiastically raised at one of the Care Programme Approach (CPA) meetings.

To explain, a CPA is a national system which serves to assess, plan, support and review the services that people with complex mental health needs receive. One of the key features of the CPA is collaboration throughout the process with the person requiring the services. In cases of young people, wherever possible, their parents/carers should be involved. All of the vulnerable people involved should be treated with dignity and respect. Indeed, this process should sit very nicely with the care value base to which health professionals work - however, experiences have highlighted that this is not necessarily the case.

To illustrate, the care value base has five main features - confidentiality, equality and diversity, rights and responsibility, anti-discriminatory practice and effective communication. All workers are expected to promote the rights of their patients (service users/clients) by way of respecting the five principles.

Unfortunately, many of Ollie's disturbing experiences were the products of the little regard shown to this guiding code. I firmly believe that professionals, purportedly assisting with management of an eating disorder, should be appropriately skilled and exceptionally versed in the idiosyncrasies of the condition.

Consequently they should be more mindful of their actions and their words - practice which some members of Ollie's team appeared to struggle with. Dangerous triggers were regularly used by staff. In the context of an eating disorder, a trigger is something that will make the eating disordered person use eating disorder behaviour.

I appreciate that when someone is battling with an eating disorder anything can be a trigger - image, word or action. Indeed, I hold up my hands and admit that I am guilty of such a practice - but I am not a professional. I believe it is understandable for parents and lay people to make such errors but not professionals.

Indeed, Ollie himself raised the issue of triggers at a CPA meeting. He specifically asked that staff refrain from congratulating him on eating. Furthermore, he didn't want to hear how much he deserved the food. And last but not least, he wanted staff to stop talking about weight. He found such talk triggering and upsetting. Regrettably, the risky unsafe chat was not eliminated from the ward floor.

Inept practice also served to significantly attack Ollie's already low self-esteem. As previously mentioned, Ollie was confined to a wheelchair due to his deficient health, but this internment did not deter unaccommodating practices.

As the designated bathroom for males was not suitable for wheelchair users he was permitted to use the girls' bathroom. This particular bathroom was of ample size and space for the wheelchair, plus it had more facilities - an important shower seat for one! Alas, one member of staff, with her inimitable charm, took it upon herself to scold Ollie like a naughty little child for using the female facilities. He was totally distraught by this vilification. After all, he was instructed to use those particular facilities, details of which should have been on his personal case notes. He had already lost his dignity and independence as a consequence of his imposed immobility, but now he felt as if staff were steadily chipping away at whatever self esteem he had remaining.

Ollie's physical presence had reduced drastically throughout the illness. A visible consequence of this was the fitting - or rather non-fitting - of his clothes, particularly his trousers. Although he did wear a belt, the dire circumstances meant that it was too big to perform its function adequately. With what seemed to be a mind of their own, the trousers soon began to drop and rest mid-bottom. Rather than help Ollie find a solution to these embarrassing occurrences, some members of staff would joke, ridicule him and at times chastise him in front of his peers, adding further to his torment. The situation could have been addressed more sympathetically and appropriately than it was.

When Ollie had reached an acceptable level of physical health, he was delighted to be able to discard the wheelchair and wander around the unit without a personal minder. Unfortunately, some staff members were not aware of Ollie's new found freedom and were extremely quick to denigrate him when they witnessed him shifting around. There were other unpleasant instances that actually cemented my theories that the provision of care by many was unprofessional and inconsistent.

As per the daily norm, I visited Ollie around afternoon break time. However, as was not the norm, he greeted me with a huge, beaming and indulgent smile on his face. It was a great warming welcome. I genuinely thought that he had something quite exciting to tell me.

My joy was swiftly crushed by his raison d'être for his apparent glee. It transpired that the reason for his genial greeting was because the staff had forgotten to give him his afternoon drink of hot chocolate and snack (a landmark victory for the anorexia). I was mortified.

Ollie's care plan categorically stipulated that he had to have a high-caloried drink and snack in the afternoon, an activity which he naturally dreaded engaging with. Nonetheless, it was an essential part of his treatment and had to be carried out.

My alarm soon changed to disgust when Ollie concluded his tale with a quote from the member of staff he had mentioned the oversight to "…But it is your responsibility to remind us." Excuse me! I do not believe that an inpatient, adolescent or adult, should be responsible for the upkeep and attention to detail of their care plans. It is, and should remain so, the responsibility of the professionals. Besides, I do not know many people living with anorexia that welcome mealtimes, yet alone snack times - much of their time is dedicated to avoiding any eating situations. I feel it is true to say that mealtimes are some of the most horrific times of day for those battling with anorexia nervosa.

Generally, mealtimes for the young inpatients were something to look forward to. Every morning there was an opportunity for them to make their lunch and teatime selections from the daily menu. This practice obviously sat well within the principles of the previously mentioned care value base - allowing the young people to make decisions about the food they wished to eat helped maintain a sense of independence and dignity. However, for Ollie this decision making process was not favoured. Neither was it easy.

Imagine the scary thought processes that he went through to make his selection. Calories. Fat content. Food groups. Colour groups. And then after the ritualistic selection, the anxiety and trepidation waiting for mealtime to occur. Just imagine having to confront your greatest fear three/four times a day - and then eat it! I'm proud and relieved to say that Ollie eventually managed to cope with this, what must have been terrifying, daily ordeal. However, there were occasions when his food nightmares were unacceptably extended.

Once again, I ask you to imagine Ollie's abounding fears; the psychological turmoil embroiled with the agonising countdown to confronting the food he had painstakingly chosen. Eyes to and fro watching the clock. Sweating and shaking as time to eat drew nearer. Waiting for mealtime was like riding an emotional roller coaster for him.

Then, imagine his feelings when he was told that he wouldn't be receiving what he was expecting as the kitchen had 'run out'! He felt as if the power to the roller coaster had been swiftly cut and was plunging rapidly into a sea of panic. There were no apologies offered to Ollie, or expressions of empathy, from staff for the position he found himself in, just cold and blunt "You'll have to have something else."

The last couple of weeks of Ollie's stay in the unit were exceptionally taxing. His progress, if one can call it that, had been erratic to say the least. At one stage, Ollie was making slight progress with his measurements, but towards the end of his stay his weight plateaued and physical measurements failed to achieve the desired numbers.

Throughout his stay he frequently felt ignored, intimidated, belittled and invisible - all negative emotions which were not conducive for the development of a happy brain, emotional health and recovery from an eating disorder. All evidence to suggest that the environment was certainly not ideal for Ollie's well-being, but the anorexia seemed to like it. Subsequently, after two particularly stressful, difficult and traumatic months, and a CPA which reported his stay in the unit as 'detrimental to his recovery', my son was duly discharged from the psychiatric unit into my loving care.

Now, one would think that my elation at the news of his homecoming could not have been dulled - wrong. Of course, I was delighted. No, let me rephrase that, ecstatic. Ollie was going to be home, starting on his journey of recovery with the people that loved him. But I had one burning question around his discharge. How was I going to successfully lead him through the battlefield of recovery without the knowledge and skills required?

It is said that people who want to recover will, and recovery will be as and when the individual wants it. Ollie's condition was a hard one to grasp. Although I felt that he wanted to recover his life, the anorexia had a different plan. There were times through his treatment when Ollie had very formidably claimed that he didn't care whether or not he died. Understandably I had suspicions that the path to recovery was going to be very fraught, frustrating and distressing. As I was the only candidate for the task to affectionately support Ollie, I had to prepare myself for the mentally draining combat ahead.

5. NEW PROVINCE OF LEARNING

"...conversations that once were humorous, enlightening and thought-provoking transformed into diminutive and trivial exchanges of words - no sentiment or feeling so as to avoid what the anxious parent really wanted to talk about."

When an eating disorder invades your home everything changes. Relationships. Routines. Roles. Nothing can truly prepare you for the turbulent times and extreme frustration lying in wait...except a little bit of awareness and understanding of the body-corrupting psychological condition.

Being so armed can provide the confidence required to challenge the eating disorder and less frightening to exude. Unfortunately, I soon discovered that I was not the only one needing to be educated about eating disorders.

Family members, armed only with society's erroneous views of eating disorders, somewhat overnight became members of the hatches, matches and despatches brigade, only caring to make contact or speak when there was a family do.

Friends suddenly became noticeable by their absence. And of those that stayed, conversations that once were humorous, enlightening and thought-provoking transformed into diminutive and trivial exchanges of words - no sentiment or feeling so as to avoid what the anxious parent really wanted to talk about - the vile antagonist in the house, the eating disorder.

In an attempt to raise awareness of the malicious anorexia that was defiling my son, I tried to encourage my family and friends to undertake a little light reading on the subject matter. I hoped that, through available texts and personal narrative, people dear to me would find a pathway to enlightenment to counter their arguments and also dispel the stigma propagating the misconceptions that they so closely held.

I must admit, I found the reading both fascinating and invaluable, especially the historical texts. Researching bygone experiences and accounts enabled me to review my beliefs about eating disorders - and most certainly helped me renounce the ubiquitous contemporary misconceptions.

No, eating disorders are not a contemporary social phenomena. Scrolls from early Chinese dynasties make references to ailments not dissimilar to today's eating disorders. Ancient Egyptian hieroglyphics illustrate the purging ritual that was practiced in order to avoid illnesses. It is even reputed that Queen Cleopatra had an obsession with her weight, so much so that she demonstrated bulimic tendencies. [5&6]

Eating disorders know no boundaries - including religion. During Medieval Europe, Western Christianity was abound with 'miraculous maidens' and their holy anorexia. This prevalence of female fasting across the continent was hugely associated with religion, with penance for sin being a major reason.

It was common custom for these extremely devout women to severely deny themselves any comforts of life. They would take to wearing clothes made of hair that were so harsh that the skin would blister. Furthermore, they would wear heavy chains and blight their bodies with self-lashing scars. Such abstemious behaviours were considered irrefutable means of cleansing one's spirit and, as such, holy maidens were held in high esteem by the Church. [7&8]

Eating disorders are not just a female issue. One of the most enlightening pieces from the annals of eating disorder history is the story of Dr Richard Morton, an established physician of the late 1600s. Despite Morton being widely recognised as an expert in the field of pulmonary disease, he is accredited with the first medical acknowledgement of anorexia nervosa.

Morton wrote about two medical cases, a sixteen-year old male student and an eighteen-year old female. The male, the son of a reverend who was a friend of Morton's, was reported to have lost his appetite for no apparent reason. Morton believed that one of the reasons for the young man's condition was his diligence to studies.

After due consideration, Morton recommended that the young man cease his studies and move to the countryside to benefit from the open air. Furthermore, he advised an asses' milk diet and horseriding as light exercise. It may seem remarkable today, but the young man's physical demeanour recovered.

The case regarding the eighteen-year old female provided a less happy conclusion. The young woman had been ill for two years with issues around appetite suppression before Morton's involvement. Sadly, she died three months later.

Morton referred to his work with these young people as cases of 'nervous consumption'. Furthermore, he strongly believed in the tenets of recovery through environment, adequate diet and moderate exercise - not unlike the mantras of today's well-being gurus. Morton's work, even centuries ago, evidenced that eating disorders knew no gender barriers.[9]

Scouring texts from books and websites was tremendously useful, but the most powerful learning tool for me was the lived experiences shared by other mothers of eating disordered children. I felt privileged to be part of this particular sisterhood. The struggles and challenges relayed by these women certainly eased my feelings of dismay and isolation.

Although I had gained a great deal of knowledge from various domains which assisted in helping me understand the intensity of anorexia and other eating disorders, it wasn't enough. I craved more.

I needed supporting theory to be able to piece together the massive jigsaw of what anorexia was.

My responsibilities at home no longer allowed me leave of absence. Therefore, any studying had to be flexible and on my own terms. Consequently, I enrolled onto an online eating disorders diploma course. The course was well structured. It contained a reasonable amount of information about particular eating disorders, but my interest was absorbed by the focus on issues around self-perception, control and responsibility, as well as the inner child. My thirst for a theoretical knowledge had been somewhat satisfied.

But it wasn't only an expansion of knowledge I required - I quickly discovered that I needed to develop my communication skills. Speaking to someone with anorexia can be frustrating and exasperating. I specifically found Ollie's all-or-nothing and personalising thought processes highly testing and upsetting. However, not speaking to an eating disordered individual in the correct manner can also be dangerous.

My feeble attempts at trying to speak to Ollie without causing friction, generating foul moods or inciting triggering situations needed to be addressed. Again, because of the very little Debbie time I now had, I trawled the internet for a further online course, one which would enhance my communication skills to support my daily responsibilities.

I enrolled on a counselling skills course which explored motivational interviewing skills. Although I was aware of motivational interviewing techniques, to actually accrue an in-depth knowledge of how such techniques help the person enabled me to respond more effectively when speaking with Ollie, and make me feel happier that I was doing everything I could to prevent harmful, traumatic, triggering episodes.

When your own child has an eating disorder, I feel that normal parenting responsibilities are terribly strained, or perhaps possibly void. I don't think that I can emphasise strongly enough just how important it is to spend time learning about the destructive eating disorder and developing relevant new skills for the new role as fundamental carer for an eating disordered child.

6. CRIPPLING CO-MORBIDS

"He would hunch his back and curl his body inwards to desperately find the folds

of repulsive fat."

Many of us experience episodes of disordered eating at some time in our lives - dieting for a Summer holiday on the beach, or bingeing on a tub of chocolates at Christmas. However, not all of us experience an eating disorder.

In order for the distinction to be determined, a diagnosis has to be made. The criteria upon which healthcare professionals worldwide base the diagnosis is found on the pages of the Diagnostic and Statistical Manual of Mental Disorders (DSM).

First published in 1952, the DSM details a number of eating disorders but it does not provide any information or guidance for the treatment of them - just straightforward matter-of-fact criteria. Of course there are many reasons for this, which include acceptance of cultural contexts and individual clinical presentations.

According to the DSM, anorexia nervosa is characterised by three main features, all of which were clearly evident in my son's experiences. These features are: intense fear of becoming fat or gaining weight; refusal to maintain body weight within the normal healthy range and body image disturbance. The body image distortion can range from someone feeling excessively overweight to others feeling that whilst they may be thin, parts of their body may be fat - hence the use of extreme measures to address their perceived 'fat' areas. [10]

Ollie had a little pastime where he employed a number of practices to evidence his so-called areas of fat. He would examine his body on the search for the ever present body padding. He would hunch his back and curl his body inwards to desperately find the folds of repulsive fat. He also used to stand upright and menacingly pull at areas of his midriff and argue that the held body mass was fat, which it clearly wasn't.

An over preoccupation with food also develops, which is a terribly demoralising and soul destroying experience for all of the family; cognitive inflexibility and inclination to avoid social events and gatherings, particularly where food might be available. Indeed this aspect of the condition can also be attributed to a condition called anhedonia. Anorexia sees the reward system of the brain severely affected which results in loss of interest in things such as food and social contact.[11]

Furthermore, self-deprecating comments and the need for approval may accompany the endeavour for perfection. I can recall how Ollie used to make constant, critical and disparaging comments about his facial features. The shape of his eyes. The size of his nose. Despite my various counter replies, nothing could sway him from his negative opinion. Even to this day, travelling the road to recovery, he remains determined to seek surgery to 'improve' his nose.

For the benefit of those readers with concerns about females - prior to the latest publication of DSM-5 in 2013, the absence of menstrual cycles was required before a diagnosis of anorexia nervosa could be given. However, this is no longer the case.

It has been recognised that pre-menarchal and post-menopausal females may develop the psychological condition, as well as those using oral contraceptives. Furthermore, the condition can also be found in women continuing to experience menstrual activity.

Although my passion was to find out all I could about anorexia, I did examine the listed criteria for bulimia nervosa and binge eating disorder. Bulimia nervosa is generally characterised by recurrent episodes of binge eating, which is accompanied by a great deal of shame, guilt and a feeling of lack of control about the behaviour.[10]

This bingeing is then followed by drastic compensatory behaviour to purge the body of the calories consumed, which includes practices such as self-induced vomiting, excessive exercise, use of laxatives and diuretics. The binge eating episodes and associated compensatory behaviours only need to occur once a week to meet the criteria for a diagnosis.

With regards to tell-tale signs, there may not be any drastic weight changes as per someone with the advanced stages of anorexia. People living with bulimia are generally normal or overweight. However there may be physical signs such as swollen glands (also referred to as 'chipmunk cheeks'). Other characteristics to be mindful of include body image disturbance, preoccupation with food, fear of becoming fat and the secret hoarding of food.

There are numerous health implications for those living with bulimia which include dental problems, gastric ruptures, rectal prolapses and oesophageal tears. Females may experience menstrual irregularity or even loss.

Prior to DSM-5, binge eating disorder was not acknowledged as an eating disorder in its own right. Similar to the condition bulimia nervosa, binge eating disorder is characterised by recurrent episodes of binge eating, occurring from once a week to at least three months.

The actual bingeing episodes, which can last for more than two hours, are associated with three or more of the following characteristics: eating huge quantities of food although not feeling hungry; eating much more hurriedly than normal; eating until feeling uncomfortably full; eating alone, and in secret, out of embarrassment over the amount consumed; feeling ashamed, disgusted, depressed or guilty about the overeating.

Whichever features are present for the individual, there will be an overwhelming sense of lack of control. However, unlike bulimia nervosa, there is no compensatory behaviour attached. [10]

Unequivocally, I think one of the most highly frustrating issues of trying to effectively care for Ollie through his battle with anorexia was the simultaneous attention I had to award to the condition's side-kicks. Ollie, as well as the majority of other people suffering with an eating disorder, suffered accompanying mental health conditions at the same time - the co-morbid conditions.

I uncovered a great deal of research in respects of co-morbidity. Not surprisingly, co-morbidity in eating disorders is a phenomenon which applies to all social groups, including young people. Apparently, more than half of teenagers with an eating disorder experience a co-morbid condition.

Some of the common coexisting conditions are devastating and debilitating conditions in their own right and hence provide a challenging task for diagnosis, treatment and recovery of eating disorders.[12]

Anosognosia

Anosognosia is probably one of the lesser acknowledged co-morbid conditions, although equally concerning. Not to be confused with denial, anosognosia is a brain-based lack of insight resulting from physical changes in the brain cells. People with this condition have no perception of their illness which leads them to acknowledge their behaviours and experiences as perfectly normal - despite others showing extreme concern for their welfare.

Consider a person battling with anorexia. As has been discussed, the effects of malnourishment on the psychological and physical being are greatly debilitating - cognitive disruption, organ damage, fatigue and weakness.

However, should that eating disordered person also be affected by anosognosia there would be no recognition or concern about the serious detrimental effects of the anorexia. The individual would feel healthy and perfectly normal. Accordingly this mindset presents severe implications for treatment and recovery - if a person does not believe themselves to be ill then they will not seek the support required to make them well.[13]

Anxiety Disorders

Everyone experiences moments of anxiety. Indeed, anxiety is a very normal part of daily life - whether it is going into a job interview, having to confront a problem at work or hovering around waiting for the first date to arrive. Although the individual can experience physical, psychological and/or behavioural symptoms of anxiety, these experiences should be recognised as natural responses to either new, disliked or alien circumstances.

However, anxiety disorders are quite different. Characterised by an un-subsiding, unrelenting worry or fear, anxiety disorders interfere drastically with one's daily life.

There are numerous long-term disorders that sit under the umbrella of anxiety disorders which include panic attacks, social anxiety disorder and generalised anxiety disorder.

It is important to note that the presence of a co-morbid anxiety can actually restrict the sufferer's recovery as the 'fear' may well intrude on any therapeutic challenges.

Bipolar Disorder

According to the Royal College of Psychiatrists, bipolar disorder (previously known as manic depression) affects around 1 in every 100 adults at some point during their life.[14]

Although there are different categorisations of bipolar disorder, those living with the condition will experience the same mood affecting characteristics, namely low and lethargic depressive states to high and overactive manic states. It is said that episodes of such extremes can last for weeks, and some may not even experience periods of 'normality' in between the swings.

Numerous studies have identified the commonality with eating disorders and bipolar, and although people with anorexia nervosa are at risk of suffering with bipolar as a co-existent condition, those living with bulimia and binge eating disorder are at a greater risk of developing the condition.

Body Dysmorphia

Body dysmorphia, also referred to as body dysmorphic disorder, is a psychological condition where the sufferer focuses on a perceived personal defect or flaw, quite usually something that no-one else can see. People living with this condition may become extremely distressed about one particular part of their body, so much so that they will seek cosmetic treatment for the offending imperfection. I have previously referred to Ollie's practice of self-deprecating remarks and his obsession with his nose.[15]

The distress and anxiety created may cause them to not want to see other people and effectively become prisoners in their own homes. Furthermore, they may spend considerable amounts of time before a mirror, giving the impression to others of vanity or self-obsession. Conversely, some may avoid mirrors altogether. Preoccupation with the distorted view of themselves not only causes great distress, but also becomes so insufferable for some that suicide is felt to be the only way out of the condition.

Borderline Personality Disorder

Borderline personality disorder (BPD) is not a common disorder, believed only to affect less than 1 percent of the population. BPD is characterised by unstable moods and emotions, self-destructive and risky behaviour, fear of abandonment or rejection, an insecure sense of identity, self harming practices and the experience of hallucinations and or delusions.

As with people living with HPD, BPD sufferers have problems forming and retaining close relationships. As can be realised, all of the mentioned characteristics can have a significant detrimental effect on daily life. The condition is found more commonly in people with bulimia and those with binge/purging anorexia and its most prominent feature is one of extremely low self-esteem. [16]

Dependent Personality Disorder

Dependent personality disorder appears in the top four co-morbid personality disorders for anorexia and bulimia, but not for those living with binge eating disorder.

In terms of characteristics, individuals with this condition constantly demean themselves, giving themselves no praise or recognition for their own skills, knowledge, abilities or judgement. Rather than praising such personal qualities and attributes they become helpless and inferior - choosing to present an over-reliance on others for decisions and guidance.[17]

Furthermore, they fear rejection and separation, particularly from individuals upon whom they depend. This in turn may subject them to experiences of abandonment, depression and isolation anxiety.

Depression

Depression is a very common mood disorder with three recognised levels - mild, moderate and severe. Some of the main features of depression are lethargy, weepiness, sadness, sleep problems, irritability and eating problems (either eating too much or appetite loss).

As with many other multi-faceted mental illnesses, the experience of depression will differ from person to person. People living with an eating disorder may experience depression as a consequence of the eating disorder or conversely experience depression prior to the onset of the eating disorder.[18]

As well as the widely known conditions of anxiety, depression and obsessive compulsive disorders, young people are particularly susceptible to developing accompanying personality disorders such as histrionic personality disorder and borderline personality disorder.

Histrionic Personality Disorder

Histrionic personality disorder (HPD) claimed to be a common co-morbid condition for those living with an eating disorder, is generally characterised by intense emotionality and excessive attention seeking behaviour, and is said to be conducive to the development of an eating disorder.[19]

It is said that someone with this disorder may be observed as being rather shallow and superficial, much preferring to engage in sexually provocative behaviour - not only to draw attention to themselves, but to also fulfil a longing for excitement and avoid routine - rather than have a serious, meaningful, romantic relationship.

Obsessive Compulsive Disorder

Although it is common for individuals to experience minor obsessions which are not problematic to our daily lives, those living with obsessive compulsive disorder (OCD) have very different, sometimes devastating, experiences. OCD is characterised by two factors - obsessions which are unrelenting, irrepressible thoughts and impulses <u>and</u> compulsions, the repetitive behaviour used to relieve oneself of the obsessional thoughts.[10]

This behaviour does not escape those living with an eating disorder. It is said that of those people living with anorexia, around 37 percent will have OCD and between 55 and 60 percent will experience an anxiety of some sort. The figure for those with bulimia is estimated at between 57 to 68 percent.[20]

As I personally witnessed, people with eating disorders utilise a great deal of energy in adopting ritualistic behaviour around food and eating.

As I am sure you can imagine, meal times were the most frightening of times for Ollie and some of the most tense times for me. The tension in the house was immense, particularly on the build up to meal time. Ollie had a number of rituals for meal times which had to be adhered to otherwise there would be great panic, upset and loud voices! The table had to be set accordingly with everything in its calculated place.

But the most important issue was around the timing of the meal - it had to be served within a certain timeframe and in relative darkness outside, which caused terrible problems during Summer. Every attempt to eliminate light entering the house had to be taken - all curtains and doors closed, and even the light through the small window above the kitchen door was blocked by strategically placed lap trays.

There are varying discussions around OCDs, particularly in children as risk factors to the development of eating disorders during adolescence and adulthood. Some authors have even asserted that people with anorexia are likely to have had a predisposition to acquiring the condition from a pre- existing OCD.

Self Harm

Although I discuss self harm in the following chapter, I believe it is germane to briefly mention self harm in its role as secretive sidekick. Self harm is a coping strategy for intense emotional and psychological distress - not a psychological illness.

Those that self harm attempt to quell overwhelming feelings such as fear, loneliness and despair through actions that help provide a temporary release from the emotional pain. Some may use the physical pain as a distraction from negative thoughts.

It is said that most people who self harm are inclined to be perfectionists and/or have an extreme dislike for their bodies - characteristics which can also be attributed to someone with an eating disorder.[21]

7. LIFE TURNED UPSIDE DOWN

"...several times he collapsed through exhaustion at the exercising, but he would pick himself up as if on automatic pilot and continue."

For a parent looking after a child who is battling an eating disorder, life can be a lonely, isolating and highly emotional existence. To be honest, I was frightened, alone and lost in a sea of alien emotions and utter inadequacy. I was not ready for the onslaught of tiring undertakings and conflict of life roles.

Being thrust into the role of fully blown, twenty-four seven, unskilled and ill-equipped carer was one of the most horrendously traumatic and emotional undertakings I had ever been obligated to do. At the time I was already coping with my 'black dog' - my depression. Life experiences were already taking their toll on my physical and mental health. Trying to hold on to that little piece of Debbie was quite a daily battle. But losing my identity as Mum pushed me into a further dark place.

There were times when I just wanted to end it all - the misery, pain and torment of watching my son fade into oblivion was agonising. I felt so drained and disassociated with the life I was living. I spent most of my time hiding behind of mask of okay-ness. It really was a struggle. Nonetheless, the needs of my ill son exceeded my own and I persisted with the fight with the help of medication and various talking therapies.

One of the most unbearable issues I attempted to sort out with therapy was my guilt at not recognising the signs of the developing eating disorder in my son. By attributing behaviour normally associated with youths and their teenage angst, my unawareness, or call it ignorance, had caused the demise of my son's adolescence - years he simply was not going to regain. The remorse I felt was intensely nauseating and extremely debilitating.

The remainder of this chapter provides a snapshot of experiences of what I now recognise as being vital clues to the enemy in the home - anorexia.

Academic Performance

Academic performance can be greatly affected by an eating disorder. Poor nutrition affects cognitive functioning which, for a young person, can have detrimental implications for school and educational studies. All through school, Ollie was an extremely conscientious, hard-working and gifted pupil, and his high attainment record didn't go without notice. At a parents' evening, Ollie's form teacher suggested that he sit his 11-plus exams for entry into one of Plymouth's high schools for boys - an invitation I chose to decline, on personal ideological grounds.

It is not uncommon for a young person with an eating disorder to promote themselves as the model student - meticulous in presentation and attention to detail; pushing themselves to achieve the highest grades. It is interesting to note academic suggestions that perfectionism contributes to the development and maintenance of eating disorders.

According to Herrin and Matsumoto, "The tendency to live by unreasonably high standards is well known to increase risk of eating disorders...when a perfectionistic child is placed in a high-pressure environment, that risk is compounded." [22] However, this drive for perfectionism could open the student up to failure, disappointment and feelings of rejection, which in some cases could lead to the onset of depression (if it is not already a presenting condition).

Conversely, due to the lack of nutritional intake, poor concentration and lethargy take hold. Some students may experience a decrease in academic performance. They may not be able to focus on assignments, assessments or tasks - or even remember anything imparted to them during lessons! Eventually, absenteeism becomes favourable to attending school, regardless of the sanctions.

Ollie remained hard-working until the eating disorder began to manifest. It was not until he started opening up about his experiences at secondary school that the true extent of how cognitive functioning is damaged by anorexia was realised.

He disclosed that he found it difficult to absorb information, no matter how many times the teacher explained something. He could not associate theories and formulae, neither could he construct meaningful sentences. Obviously the constant non-compliance, albeit unintentional, with instructions and orders at school impacted upon his relationships with a few members of staff.

Many would consider his slide to inaptitude for school work as expressions of rebellion and teenage angst, when in reality it was anorexia and its attempt to consume him.

Bloatedness

Frequent complaints of bloatedness can be telling indicators of an eating disorder, particularly anorexia and bulimia. Such ailments could be due to the resulting biochemical changes that people with eating disorders experience, and the changes to regulatory signals from the brain. For example, those living with anorexia do not produce the appropriate enzymes to digest food.

However, as it was in Ollie's case, bloating can also be attributed to the excessive chewing of sugarless gum. One of the common ingredients in sugarless chewing gum is Sorbitol, known to be a substance which the body cannot absorb. The regular, and often continuous, chewing of this indigestible product causes bloating to occur.[23]

Body Checking

Although the practice of 'checking' is generally associated with obsessive compulsive disorders (which are known to be co-morbid conditions of eating disorders), people living with an eating disorder and accompanying sidekick 'body dysmorphia' will develop obsessive body checking behaviour.

Preoccupation with weight, shape, size and appearance leads to certain behaviours which may seem to present themselves as narcissistic 'acts of vanity'. Such behaviours include frequent weighing, pinching the body to identify areas of 'fat', constant measuring of body parts, seeking continuous gratifying assurance from others of their appearance and repeatedly looking at their reflection.

Initially, Ollie's body checking was one of the more difficult behaviours to contend with. No mirror or window, in fact anything that offered a reflection, was sacred to his glances. I recall that he would stand in front of the hall mirror for minutes on end inspecting his profile...and make accompanying disparaging remarks on what he saw. He couldn't walk past a stationary car without taking a sneaky peek in the wing mirror at his image.

I am ashamed to admit it but I found this body checking behaviour absolutely appalling because I associated it with vanity. Vanity is a characteristic that I have never applauded in anyone and hate to see even more so in one of my children.

Due to the distorted perception, regardless of values, personal attributes and merits that those living with eating disorders have, they will ultimately check their bodies for things they <u>do not</u> like as opposed to things they <u>do</u> like - the search for imperfections will be a never-ending journey.

Chewing Gum

Until I started researching eating disorders, I never associated gum chewing with anorexia, and Ollie obsessively chewed gum. But not any old gum - sugarless gum. As soon as one stick had been masticated a couple of hundred times, another was swiftly unwrapped and popped into his mouth. It was almost as if he was on auto-pilot.

It is a widely known fact that sugarless gum has no nutritional value and very little calorific value (a tick for the anorexic's intentions). However, what is not widely recognised is the role of brain chemistry in the gum chewing activity - particularly serotonin.

Serotonin, the neurotransmitter which increases the feeling of well-being, is produced when people chew - the more people chew the better they will feel. Chewing also leads the body to believe that food is imminent and subsequently serves to temporarily satisfy any hunger pangs. Recently sugarless gum has been promoted through the media as a convenient product for dental health. However, for someone with an eating disorder it is something more. [24]

Sugarless gum is quite often sweetened by Sorbitol, a sugar alcohol, which is not as sweet as sugar, and neither is it as calorific. However, it is also a laxative, especially when consumed excessively. Of course, any type of gum can act as an ideal concealer of unsavoury compensatory behaviour such as self-induced vomiting. [24]

Clothes

Clothes are not just about keeping warm or avoiding arrest for indecent exposure. Clothes assist in defining our identity. For many young people, clothes are the visual statement of belonging. Belonging to a peer group is central to personal and social development. It enables the young person to 'fit in' to a society which may otherwise give the impression of them being unwanted, unvalued and ignored.

It is quite common for peer groups to become the main source of advice and help, often replacing any parent and family involvement. Indeed, peer groups are known to be very powerful in not only influencing a young person's values but also preferences for sport, music and style of clothes…and style of clothing is just as important to someone with anorexia, regardless of age.

It is not uncommon for people living with anorexia to change their dress code to one of wearing baggy items for baggy clothes are valuable aids in the art of the anorexics deception.

Anorexia is a secretive illness, and the sufferer will do practically anything to keep the condition from being found out. Wearing baggy clothes, essentially those which cover the whole body, will allow the body changes to remain hidden from family, friends and colleagues for as long as viably possible - and hence permit ongoing weight loss.

Ollie became part of the Emo and Goth subculture. Within no time at all he turned his back on his Tony Hawk skater boy image and proudly donned all that was black - including the thickest eyeliner ever. I wasn't concerned about this change of direction. As a former Sociology lecturer, I was well versed in the attributes of peer groups and the rites of passage. It was a necessary part of Ollie's personal journey to independence.

Unfortunately, I didn't notice how, over time, the clothes became baggier. Even his nightwear was replaced by his older brother's big, black, baggy Top Man jumper - a jumper which had arms so long it covered Ollie's finger tips. But baggy clothes can also serve to act as security blankets for anorexics. Tight clothes, fitting snuggly against the skin, could make the anorexic feel fat, thereby fuelling the generally associated body dysmorphia.

When a change in dress code is noted it is very important to also be watchful for any accompanying accessories. As I have previously mentioned it is very rare for an eating disorder to be unaccompanied by a sidekick - and a change in dress code can equally be accompanied by deceiving accessories. For example, co-morbid self harming practices can be masked by the ever popular silicone charity wrist bands or inches of decorative bangles and bracelets.

Cold Showers

It is reported through various sources that taking cold showers assists with weight loss. It is no surprise therefore that many anorexics choose this body-shivering way to shower. Exposure to cold temperatures accelerates the metabolism as the body uses energy (from its fat store) in an attempt to keep warm. Basically, as the freezing water hits the skin, the body jolts because of the shock. Consequently, the heart rate and blood flow increase and muscles begin to harden. These metabolic processes all require energy, i.e. need to burn calories.

I have been a victim of this rather nasty little practice. On three occasions throughout the course of a month, as I turned on the shower I was furiously attacked by forceful sub-zero gushes of freezing cold water. Initially, I thought that the shower's thermostat was playing up. It didn't occur to me that Ollie had been altering the gauge to appease the anorexia.

Condiments

Ollie developed a ritual of smothering his food in tomato ketchup. It wasn't until I started researching the complexities of anorexia nervosa that I recognised this behaviour as a notable trait of the condition. Whilst it is common practice for those with anorexia to promote condiments to the realm of food group status, their excessive condiment use can be suitably referred to as condiment abuse.

The two most common ways of practicing condiment abuse is 1) when food is smothered so much with condiments that it renders food inedible, and 2) when condiments are added to incompatible food stuffs.

As previously mentioned, the art of condiment abuse did not escape Ollie. His compulsion for tomato ketchup was sometimes mortifying. He would think nothing of adding six or seven sachets of ketchup to his meal, maybe more on occasions. Believe me when I say that it was always brilliant when he managed to eat, even when smothered in tomato ketchup. For just for a few moments I would feel as if all of the world's worries had been lifted. However, learning about his addition of ketchup to his breakfast cereal was definitely not one of those finer moments.

Dental Issues

Anorexia infiltrated Ollie's once decent levels of personal hygiene - including his dental hygiene. Although not widely talked about, or even considered, eating disorders can affect oral health in a number of ways.

For a long time Ollie found it extremely difficult to engage with the dental practice. He would muster up numerous excuses to miss appointments. It wasn't until he started to open up about things that I found out he had actually developed a morbid fear of cleaning his teeth. He feared swallowing toothpaste - not because of any possible ill-health effects but because of increasing his daily calorie intake.

Alongside the possibility of developing an unsavoury smelling breath, the physical consequences of an eating disorder on the mouth can be extremely embarrassing for some:- enamel erosion (caused by the repeated contact with stomach acid through self-induced vomiting); tooth loss (which occurs due to the lack of calcium and Vitamin D, resulting in osteoporosis which affects the jaw bone); gum disease (which develops as a consequence of poor nutrition), and glossitis (inflammation of the tongue which can be caused by mineral deficiencies).

Being able to provide effective help and support for matters around oral health are equally important as other areas of support, particularly as the correlation between oral health and poor mental health is becoming more documented. Indeed, I was rather bemused that when attending CPA meetings the issue of dental care wasn't raised.

Nonetheless, throughout this whole life-changing, eating disorder experience, I have had the privilege to meet some fantastic supportive people. Frances Marriott, a former dental hygienist now an oral health educator, is one of those people.

Initially, I was oblivious to Ollie's occasional bouts of self-induced vomiting and consequently not aware of the significant damage he was doing to his teeth. However, Fran provided me with basic tips that helped me support Ollie with his oral health, which seriously made my life easier and placed my mind at a higher level of ease.

For instance, she suggested encouraging Ollie to avoid brushing his teeth after a vomiting episode but to rinse his mouth out with water instead. This was preferred as it would prevent the acceleration of enamel erosion by preventing gastric acid from being brushed directly onto his teeth.

Plus, to further protect tooth enamel, Fran recommended that Ollie used a straw when drinking a fizzy drink in order to steer the acidic beverage away from the teeth. I can assure you, it wasn't long before I had an endless supply of plastic striped straws congregating in my cupboard.

The dentist or dental hygienist could be the first health professional to uncover the manifestation of an eating disorder - well before parents and carers become aware of the despicable condition. It is therefore vitally important to ensure that regular dental checks are maintained.

Dizziness

Spells of light-headedness or dizziness are quite common indicators of general unwellness. However, dizziness can also be a sign of a dangerous presiding eating disorder which many will miss - I hold my hands up and confess fervently to being guilty of this.

Eating disorders are secret manifestations and secretive behaviours accompany them, for example compulsive exercising and intake restriction. These behaviours have a negative impact on the body and its systems, which in turn cause serious medical conditions such as low blood pressure, irregular heartbeat and dehydration.

On several occasions Ollie complained of feeling light-headed. I responded to his ailment in the way one would in generally healthy people - advising him to take a moment of composure and fluid intake increase. If only I had known about his secret illness.

Eating disorders don't like being found out, and like being tackled and manipulated even less. Ollie became a very restless and agitated young man, always needing to be on the go and burning calories. Sitting still meant less expenditure of calories which the anorexia didn't welcome.

Drinks

The benefits of adequate daily fluid intake for the body are immense.

Fluids, whether water or as found in foods, help energise muscles, keep bowels and kidneys functioning and maintain body temperature. It is essential therefore that fluids, which are lost as a matter of course through normal bodily functions such as breathing and sweating, are replaced. If the lost fluid is not replaced the body will become dehydrated.

Dehydration affects the body in numerous ways - irritability, constipation, headaches, kidney stones. Unfortunately, life-conserving health-sustaining fluids are not always regarded with esteem by some living with an eating disorder.

Some with eating disorders will turn to artificial substances in an attempt to either gain more energy or suppress their appetite and hence achieve a feeling of fullness. It is not uncommon therefore for anorexics to consume numerous energy drinks or copious amounts of black coffee.

Caffeine, one of the substances present in both drinks, is a widely available mild diuretic. Diuretics are substances which promote urine production and are frequently used by those living with an eating disorder in an attempt to lose weight.

Remuda Ranch, a hospital for eating disorders in America, makes an interesting observation in that people with eating disorders actually confuse the effect of temporary fluid loss with actual weight loss. [25]

Caffeine consumption can also develop into an addiction as well as have some serious health consequences, particularly for those living with an eating disorder. Ollie was a tea drinker like me. He never used to drink coffee so I must admit to being a little shocked when he asked for his first cup of coffee at home. In the early days, Ollie drank his coffee white, with a splash of skimmed milk. But, as the undercover anorexia progressed, the drop of milk became too challenging. Ollie eventually became a devout consumer of black coffee and protested profusely if I inadvertently added milk - his reactions were fierce as if I had tried to poison him.

Regrettably, water is also used as an appetite suppressant and as a convenient means to providing the sensation of fullness. In addition, it is a very useful tool for deceit. I recall Ollie went through a phase of drinking abundant amounts of water before his GP appointments - the term used for this is 'water loading'. He wanted to give the impression that his weight had increased. This would prevent any GP interrogations and therefore reduce any further interference by the health professionals. However, 'water loading' can also have serious consequences for the individual such as electrolyte imbalance and cardiac arrest.

No sugar, low calorie cordials and fizzy drinks are also favourites of those with eating disorders - which my son avidly evidenced. However, these drinks, whilst serving to appease the calorie conscious conditions, are also initiators of physical inflictions. The artificial sweeteners commonly used in such drinks can cause ailments such as diarrhoea, bloating and extreme abdominal pain.

Excessive (Compulsive) Exercising

I recall how one day, long before the dreaded diagnosis, Ollie excitedly told me that he had just done one hundred star jumps. His face beamed in his success. I was really pleased for him and inside I rejoiced. His days of sitting in front of the PlayStation were coming to an end. My youngest child was growing up. Unfortunately, it was only as things unfurled that I realised my role in the eating disorder's malicious attack on my son.

Although it must be acknowledged that exercise plays an important role in a healthy lifestyle, which should not be discouraged, it is possible that some may pursue excessive exercise regimes for adverse reasons.

Someone with an eating disorder may purposely use exercise as a purging tool to eliminate unwanted calories. Such erroneous thinking cannot only have a detrimental effect on a person's quality of life, but can place them at risk of acquiring a severe injury. The compulsive thoughts can even result in the eating disordered person exercising in secret. For Ollie this meant rigorous clandestine activity in the privacy of his bedroom late at night. Not many weeks after his diagnosis he revealed his sacred practice of three hundred star jumps a night. Guilt dealt me a body blow - hard.

Following his disturbing disclosure I was stunned. I didn't know what to do, how to play it. I was aware at this stage that any attempts to interrupt, prevent or stop the exercising could trigger extreme anxiety, mood swings and even hostility.

Nonetheless, accepting that my already sleepless nights were about to become more extreme I would lay in bed every night with one ear rested down on the pillow and the other finely tuned into the room above. I couldn't afford to sleep for Ollie's sake.

Reflecting, I think one of the most shocking discoveries associated with the anorexia afflicting my son was when I walked in on him in the kitchen as he was performing star jumps!

Ollie was in full exertion mode, back straight against the unit, sternly front facing the wall in the corner of the kitchen. A gentle thud accompanied the dramatic flapping of his bony arms. With what appeared to be great determination he managed to turn his head to face me. Tears were streaming down his cheeks. Desperately he called out, "Mum, help, I can't stop. I can't stop. Help." He literally could not stop. The longer he star-jumped, the more tears he shed - and I with him. It took what seemed an eternity to be able to coax him to stop.

This compulsion for excessive exercise will see the person exercise as if on automatic pilot, regardless of pain, injury or harm to self. It is known that some will exercise far beyond the limits to their health, for instance, ignoring any fractures or strains, tendon or muscle injuries. To my horror, Ollie divulged that on numerous occasions he collapsed through exhaustion at the uncontrollable exercising.

Feeling Cold

Ollie was always complaining of feeling cold, even on days of glorious sunshine. Quite often he would wrap himself in his zebra print snuggle (blanket with sleeves) and welcome the endless stream of hot water bottles. The central heating would be switched on, sometimes simultaneously with the gas fire in the lounge, but to no avail - he remained chilled to the bone, as the saying goes. The type of cold Ollie was experiencing was not the general peripheral cold air but the endogenous circumstances of anorexia. His restrictive intake practices were affecting his body's fat store - his body's insulation. The less he ate over time, the more of his body tissue and reserves he lost. This in turn impacted on the amount of heat his body could generate. Quite simply - no fuel no heat!

Hair

No part of the body escapes the effects of an eating disorder. Some consequences are internal and therefore are only uncovered when the medical professionals begin scaled tests and monitoring.

However, one of the more visible signs is the change in the condition of someone's hair. Despite someone with anorexia drinking bountiful amounts of low-calorie drinks, it is not sufficient to keep the body hydrated.

Due to dehydration and lack of vitamin and mineral intake, hair becomes brittle and lifeless, often falling out when touched. Indeed, it was not uncommon for Ollie's hair to come out in little clumps as he ran his hands through it.

Also, as a result of malnutrition, starvation and lack of body fat, anorexics will find a soft, downy hair growing on their bodies called lanugo. Derived from the Latin *lanugo down* (lana "wool"), lanugo normally associated with new-born babies grows in an attempt to keep itself warm.

Lanugo acts like a personal heated blanket for the anorexic. Although generally found to grow on the face, back and arms, it has been known to grow all over the body. Ollie developed lanugo hair on his face and chest. However, once his nutritional recovery began, the hair disappeared.

Hands

Under anorexia, the body experiences substantial pressure where no part of the anatomy is sacred - this includes the heart. As the heart loses mass, its ability to perform as normal is affected. Heart rate decreases and so does blood pressure - a consequence of these changes is poor circulation. Whilst these features are taking place on the inside, there are very visible signs externally.

Hands, and other protrusions, become very cold and turn blue, almost purple in some cases. Many people with anorexia develop a common condition called Raynaud's disease (or phenomenon). Generally, this condition is triggered by extremes of cold weather, however the circulatory problems experienced by those with anorexia can materialise at any time. Ollie was diagnosed with Raynaud's. To manage the condition he had an exceptional supply of fingerless gloves.

Low self-esteem

Self-esteem is generally described as the way in which we value ourselves. When someone is experiencing low self-esteem it is not uncommon for them to adopt coping mechanisms to help them deal with their daily lives, including eating disorders.

Young people are particularly susceptible to developing low self-esteem. Indeed, there are a number of factors that may contribute to a young person's feeling of worthlessness and eventual deterioration in self-esteem. These factors include bullying, teasing, name calling whether by peers or family members. Consequently, any young person holding such negative opinions of themselves may not cope as well at those with positive self-esteem when faced with stressful and profound family matters such as divorce, moving house and loss of a loved one.

According to the charity YoungMinds, children and young people with low self-esteem will have a negative image of themselves; feel bad, ugly, unlikeable or stupid; lack confidence; find it hard to make and keep friendships; feel victimised by others; tend to avoid new things and find change hard and also tend to put themselves down.[26]

One of the features of low self-esteem is self-deprecation - the constant verbal devaluing of the self. Someone experiencing low self-esteem may make negative remarks about themselves and their abilities; may comment about people wasting time, money and energy on them and overtly reject any compliments.

I recollect the numerous destructive comments my son used to make with reference to not only his features, but his appearance, skills and knowledge. This mode of talk wasn't the occasional one-off remark, it was the constant dripping of downbeat disapproval of himself. Not only does such negative self-talk help perpetuate the cycle of devaluation and loss of self-worth, it also affects loved ones.

To hear your child incessantly talk themselves down is heartbreaking, particularly when you see the opposite of what is being spouted. When you can visualise a future and they a bleakness. When you realise that there is so much hurt and self-despise that your love alone isn't going to be able to achieve much (if anything) to make them feel better about themselves, that is heartbreaking.

Low self-esteem provokes self-deprecating destructive practices, such as 'fat talk' - negative body talk, which gives the eating disorder a dangerous platform. Unfortunately, this unconstructive practice cleverly exploits the words of others for the eating disorder's delight. I had to be mindful of my own 'fat talk'. Not that I did it very often but, due to the manner in which comments about food and weight issues are absorbed and twisted by the eating disorder, I did not want Ollie to add further focus to his already distorted perceptions. Indeed, one of the most helpful things for someone with an eating disorder is to have contact with body positive individuals throughout their lives.

Whenever possible, I talked with Ollie about his personal qualities, attributes and values. All in the hope that somewhere along the journey he would recognise that one's worth is not about what someone looks like but what they are like as a person.

Moodiness

As mentioned in an earlier section of this book, Ollie was a happy, friendly little boy. But, like so many young adults, in his teenage years he became partial to the customary adolescent mood swing strop - or at least that is what I believed then. My research into eating disorders presented me with a different area of consideration.

There is a particular complex system of the body which plays a significant role in eating disorders and that is the Hypothalmic-

Pituitary-Adrenal Axis (HPA) system.[27]

This HPA system is connected with three areas of the brain - the hypothalamus, pituitary gland and the amygdala, and it produces the chemicals that regulate appetite, mood and stress. When the production of these neurotransmitters is affected, as seen in someone with anorexia nervosa, then mood swings are experienced. Ollie was in the throes of anorexia in his teenage years. This malfunctioning system could have been a contributory factor for his outbursts.

Nails

Although fingernails and toenails may appear to be an unusual casualty of anorexia, they are in fact, very good indicators of the existence of the malicious condition. As with hair, nails become brittle and fragile. Indeed, Ollie often reported on how he could easily rip his nails.

Furthermore, nails could experience certain discolouration for a variety of reasons. Nails become blue and discoloured as a result of poor circulation. Malnutrition may cause noticeable ridges to develop. The lack of calcium and vitamins A and D causes brittleness, and the lack of iron can result in spoon-shaped nails. Also, as a consequence of low albumin levels, albumin being the protein which provides the body with the protein required to sustain growth and tissue repairs, nails may turn yellow.

Obsession with Numbers

It is not uncommon for someone with an eating disorder to be preoccupied with numbers, any numbers. This behaviour can be found across all areas of daily life - whether it's commenting on dress sizes or eyeing up the calorie content on food packets. In actual fact, supermarket shopping with Ollie whilst in the early stages of treatment and recovery, was one of the activities I dreaded the most. Not because the shopping visit would be extended by nearly three times the duration, but because of how others viewed him.

To the unaware, Ollie's scrutiny of food packets would be considered somewhat odd and unorthodox behaviour. If he didn't pick up an item for close meticulous inspection then he would simply stand motionless and read the label of every product on the shelf in front of him - which included items in the chilled section. Not a fun pastime. Shoppers would walk back and forth along the aisle, giving an occasional glare towards my son's direction and even childishly whisper to their partners.

Of course Ollie was oblivious to the machinations of the fellow consumers. He was solely occupied with tending to his obsession - his need to count calories. Alongside the calorie counting tribulations of supermarket shopping was the routine - the ritual of traipsing up and down the aisles. Ollie had set himself a routine.

The aisles of the supermarket had to be explored in exactly the same order for every visit. If this was not possible, for whatever reason, Ollie's anxiety would heighten. The tension would increase dramatically as he hovered around, waiting for the opportunity to continue with his personal custom. Needless to say, this added further despair to the shopping experience.

Personal Hygiene

It is known that psychological conditions, such as depression, can affect an individual's attention to personal hygiene - and this can also be the case for someone with an eating disorder. For many psychological disorders, the interest in personal hygiene may wane due to a total lack of interest and motivation. However for someone with anorexia, this issue could be more to do with the accompanying body dysmorphic disorder.

As mentioned in a previous chapter, body dysmorphic disorder is a psychological condition associated with an obsessive preoccupation with a perceived abnormality in appearance, which in some cases can be life-threatening. Reluctance to wash or shower emanates from being unable to look at or touch their own body. Shower gel and the nice smelly gift sets for Christmas or birthdays were a definite no-no for Ollie. His utter dislike for his body impacted greatly on his ability and motivation to shower. In his own mind's eye he could see the 'rolls of fat' and hence couldn't bear to touch his own body.

Ollie also experienced extreme periods of bad, fruity-smelling breath called ketosis - quite common in those living with the extreme effects of anorexia. Ketosis happens when the body is no longer able to burn carbohydrates for energy, but instead burns body fat. As the fat is converted it creates chemicals called ketones. It is these ketones that cause the unpleasant smell. This, alongside his fear of cleaning his teeth, was extremely difficult to deal with - particularly as I feared how he would cope with the effect of any outbreak of infections as a result of his poor hygiene.

Preoccupation with Food

For a person either with or developing an eating disorder, regardless of which type, food and food-related material becomes the most important focus of their life. The obsession presents itself in a multitude of ways. However, there is a very good reason why food preoccupation becomes an enormous feature in the lives of so many living with an eating disorder, in particular, anorexia nervosa.

On reading, I have found that there are a number of hormones which affect our hunger, appetite and feeding. I would like to specifically focus on the hormones, Ghrelin, Leptin and Orexin.

Ghrelin is a stomach produced hormone which is released in vast amounts before eating. It promotes food intake by signalling to the brain that the body 'wants' food. The longer the body waits to be fed, the level of Ghrelin increases. After eating Ghrelin levels fall.

Leptin, a previously mentioned hormone which is released into the blood by fat cells, is an appetite suppressant and inhibitor of food intake. When we eat, Leptin sends signals to the hypothalamus (part of the brain responsible for hunger) when the body has had sufficient to eat, i.e. the feeling of satiety (fullness). Together these two hormones work as a balancing act for our hunger.[28]

However, when we do not eat, the brain performs a trick to assist in finding food for ourselves. Our ancestors needed to be able to hunt even though their bodies' energy supplies were dwindling. Finding food at this stage could mean the difference between life and death.[29] It is for this very reason that the brain releases a hormone known as Orexin.

Orexin is a relatively new hormone known to us which is responsible for, among other things, generating the desire to 'actively search for food'. But Orexin also inhibits the appetite suppressant Leptin which subsequently leads to the most overwhelming and powerful food cravings. An anorexic's preoccupation with food could rightly be apportioned to the lack of food intake creating exceptional hormonal changes in the body.[30]

Ollie demonstrated his preoccupation with food in a multitude of ways:-

Books and literature - We would often visit the local charity shops and whilst I would busy myself around the clothes rails, Ollie would stand and salivate over the cookery books. More often than not, he would purchase one, two, even three.

He was also an avid collector of free recipe cards from the supermarkets and menus from cafés and pubs. Endlessly, he would trawl the internet for titillating food images and write recipe books - not for him of course, for others. But it didn't stop there. He even submitted his own recipe for a vegetarian Sea Bed sandwich to an online student recipe site.

Cooking and baking - Prior to Ollie's diagnosis, I would never ever have associated the desire to bake or cook with a fatal psychological illness. But it's true. Endless streams of personal narrative by people living with anorexia discuss the enjoyment of creating wonderful cakes and meals.

People living with anorexia get remote pleasure in watching people eat. By saying no to the calories; not succumbing to temptation; denying oneself a treat due to notions of being 'undeserving of nice things', a sense of being in control is experienced - and enjoyed. I remember how keen Ollie was to help prepare meals, make sandwiches, even sort out breakfast.

Initially, I thought his interest to help me was to combat his boredom - but I was wrong. I was truly amazed at how well he could just throw food together and end up with the tastiest concoction ever...and his baking! Wow!

Ollie made the most scrumptious, light and airy cakes in the world - my mouth is watering now at the thought of those delectable delights...and the great fervour in which he decorated his baking accomplishments was astounding. He applied such care and attention to his creations. Slowly, and with great precision, he would place the edible adornments on his freshly baked treats. Each item looked as good as it tasted. Of course, Ollie never tasted any of his masterpieces. He would become extremely upset if I didn't want to eat any of his feats - and I now know why.

Ollie used to show an intense interest in my partaking of a slice of cake. His whole face would light up with extreme pleasure as I sank my teeth into the yummy morsel - it was as if he was eating the cake with me, getting his 'fix' for want of a better word, which, based on the research I have conducted, he was. My son was merrily inveigling me to consume multitudes of calories a time for his, what seems to be now, perverse pleasure.

Television programmes - I think Ollie's obsession with 'food TV' was one of the hardest features for the family to deal with - it almost drove us apart.

It wasn't the self-promotion to 'Master of the Remote Control', it was more his uncanny ability to sniff out food-related programmes like a bloodhound and surreptitiously become affixed to the screen as if his life depended on it.

But his commandeering of the television did not stop at food programmes and their repeats an hour later. His obsession infiltrated all programmes - even my beloved Countdown, the longest running television game show in the world.

I used to look forward to grabbing five minutes' respite from my caring duties - sat in front of the television, cup of tea in hand, embracing the opportunity to challenge my grey matter with the boggling disciplines of letters, numbers and nine-letter anagrams.

However, it didn't take long before Ollie crowned himself top lexicographer…for finding food-related words in the contestant's letter selection, every single time!

Purging

Purging is the compensatory activity for relieving the body of unwanted calories. This extreme method of weight control is performed in a variety of ways, for example:- through self-induced vomiting, excessive exercise and the use of laxatives (which work by stimulating the bowel muscles). Furthermore, if laxatives are used regularly, the bowel muscles cease working by themselves thus creating a dependency.

Although purging is a common feature of bulimia nervosa, some with anorexia can also be prone to the practice. As previously mentioned, my son participated in excessive compulsive exercise and also self-induced vomiting. On occasions, I would find suspect dark stains and residue in the sink basin. Being rather naive and unaware of Ollie's purging practices, I just cleaned the offending presence away. I do feel rather ridiculous and ashamed now that I never thought to question Ollie about my findings at the time.

Purging, as well as being ineffective, has serious, highly dangerous consequences for the body. Self-induced vomiting can cause the erosion of tooth enamel to the rupturing of the oesophagus. Electrolytes in the body can become unbalanced and cause heart problems.

Restlessness

Many people living with anorexia often experience hyperactivity. As mentioned in an earlier section, this can be the result of low levels of Leptin which can incite an inability to relax. Another explanation could be the behavioural characteristics of some co-morbid conditions such as heightened anxiety, where exercise might be used as a channel to eliminate any negative feelings.

There are numerous inappropriate fidgety behaviours of which Ollie adopted quite a few. For example, he would sit and make his leg continuously tremble by placing pressure on the ball of his foot. Regardless of his aching joints, poor circulation and other mobility problems, the anorexia would not allow him to rest, promoting walking as the preferred pastime.

Knowing the delicate state of Ollie's heart, I found it very difficult not to worry about his lengthy walking pursuits. His condition meant that he could collapse at any time. Needless to say my worry turned into fear when he candidly mentioned to me that quite often, as a result of his insomnia and compulsion to exercise, he sneaked out of the house in the early hours to walk around the grounds of the local park.

Self harm

Very rarely are eating disorders seen as issues of self harm - but they are. The damaging restrictions and rituals that people with eating disorders impose upon themselves do harm to the body and also the mind.

People self harm in a variety of ways which can be via direct or indirect methods. It may be pertinent to think of an eating disorder as having a slow, trickle effect upon the individual.

Key underlying features of an eating disorder are poor body image and low self-esteem. Feelings of guilt, anger, shame and self-loathing may be so intense in this group of people that they may carry out self-inflicted physical pain as a coping strategy, rather than deal with their deep emotional pain. Some may use self harm as a form of self-punishment for not adhering to the self-imposed routines, i.e. not fulfilling quota on star jumps (another of Ollie's behaviours).

Much to my dismay, Ollie disclosed how he occasionally managed his emotional turmoil through cutting and burning himself, quite direct methods of self harm - however, this declaration was not a total surprise to me. I had spotted the occasional fragment of mirror on the floor of his bedroom but, being so naive and ignorant, I didn't think anything other than he had broken something and had created a bit of a shambles trying to clean it up. I know now that I should have approached him about my findings - I was just oblivious to the whole picture.

Ordinarily when people hear the phrase self harm, the usual practices that enter thoughts are of cutting and burning. These are very common practices, particularly for those with binge-purging tendencies.

However, the list of self harming methods is less exhaustive than you may realise. Other practices include the ingestion of toxic materials, hitting and punching body parts, head banging, interference with wounds and alcohol and substance abuse.

Some key visual and behavioural indicators for self harm include: constant bruising; claims to have had an accident; carrying a lighter when a non-smoker; wearing long sleeved clothes in hot weather; keeping sharp items close to them. Regardless of the severity of the self harming methods used, the actions should not be mistaken as intentional attempts to complete suicide.

Sleep problems

Numerous factors are implicated in the causes of sleep problems in those with eating disorders. There are issues around electrolyte disturbances and hormonal problems; side effects of medications used to treat co-morbid conditions such as depression; and the effects of copious amounts of caffeine, either from excessive cups of coffee or energy drinks.

There is also a rather sinister explanation, one which Ollie enlightened me to - the fear of dying whilst asleep - a fear I understand was not uncommon amongst the eating disordered community. Ollie was fully aware of the severe impact that anorexia had on his body, markedly the wasting away of his heart, low blood pressure and slow heart rate, and the increased risk of cardiac arrest that they all presented. Needless to say, night time often added to his already anxious life.

Suicidal Thoughts

Eating disorders are the most fatal of psychological illnesses, with anorexia ranking highest in level of fatality. Unfortunately, the deaths are not all due to the deterioration of the body. It is commonplace for people living with anorexia to experience suicidal thoughts - with some actually colluding with the destructive thoughts.

Suicidal thoughts may emerge for a variety of reasons, such as unwillingness to take prescribed medication for either eating disorder or co-existing disorder due to possible side effects; skewed thoughts and perceptions as a consequence of the malnutrition; a history of past abuse (which is noted as a significant factor in the cause of suicide in eating disordered people) and a desperate feeling of worthlessness.

Furthermore, the methods used to attempt suicide are, in the main, quite severe, foolproof methods which indicate the overwhelming intention to succeed.

Knowing the correlation of anorexia to suicide was an intolerable strain for me. I was already watching my son slowly kill himself through self-starvation - which was unbearable enough - but the thought that he might one day take his own life, and by some chilling and gruesome means, was totally soul destroying.

There were times when I just sailed along with my son's detached emotions, trying to avoid the despair and hurt when he would say things like he didn't care about living and wanted to die. My son's regular encounters with suicidal ideation were terribly distressing moments, moments which penetrated my mind and soul. I truly cannot express strongly enough, and without pain, just how deeply it cut through the heart.

At this point I feel it pertinent to mention that I have discovered a remarkable mental health literacy course, Mental Health First Aid (MHFA).

The MHFA course covers a variety of topics including exploration of common mental health conditions, communication skills, stress buckets. Furthermore, it seeks to equip individuals with a personal toolkit of skills and knowledge which not only assist in the provision of comfort and initial support to someone experiencing mental health distress - I refer to Ollie's anxiety attacks here, but also in preserving the life of someone where there may be a danger to themselves or others - Ollie's suicidal ideation and correlated language! Had I been aware of its existence earlier, I feel that I could have been saved from the overabundance of mental anguish, fear and guilt.

The roller coaster of emotions and mental distress that we experienced during Ollie's darkest days may well have been calmed had I been able to draw on the skills and knowledge that I obtained from the course.

If there is any solace to be found from such upsetting experiences of hearing that your child wishes to no longer live, it is that suicidal thoughts are said to recede once the recovery process starts.

Unusual eating habits

In relation to anorexia, one of the most apparent tell-tale signs of a lurking or existing condition is the development of strange behaviours around food. In an attempt to restrict intake many rituals may be cunningly devised. For example, cutting food into very tiny pieces and then eating only a small amount; preferring to only eat certain coloured food; not liking different types of food touching each other on the plate.

People with bulimic tendencies will also display signs of unusual eating habits. However, the evidence might not be found via the dinner plate, but more as heaps of discarded food and sweet wrappers under the bed, in drawers and in cupboards.

Ollie had an almanac of food rituals. Some were rather intriguing to encounter whilst others were undeniably irritating to watch, such as chasing a solitary garden pea around the plate or cutting up food into the tiniest of pieces. He habitually broke up sandwiches. He would start the procedure by tearing the crusts away. He would then reassemble the filling and carefully finish the ritual by crumbling the sandwich so much that there were merely breadcrumbs on the plate.

Cheese sandwiches regularly survived such destruction. However, the grated cheese for which he had a penchant, fell out of the sandwich so frequently that it was debatable as to how much of a sandwich or simply bread he had eaten.

The most irritating of delaying tactics employed was the extremely slow and laborious manner in which he ate his food. He would take the smallest of bites, and repeatedly chew and chew and chew. Each morsel a challenge in a game which he seemed to enjoy competing in.

Ollie divulged how his behaviour towards food switched from being a conscious pastime at the dinner table to a dangerous eating diversion. Initially, he experimented with how much food he could leave on his plate - amounts of which increased over time. This once playful activity became a habit, which in turn became an obsession and then an addiction.

Vegetarianism

From personal experience, I now regard vegetarianism as a form of legitimate restrictive eating which can help mask a developing eating disorder. Indeed, there are numerous articles and studies identifying vegetarianism as a risk factor for the onset of eating disorders in young people. Some make reference to young people becoming vegetarian in order to eat more healthily, when in fact they are attempting to control their intake of high fat foods.[31]

Ollie became a self-proclaimed vegetarian at the tender age of six. His school had visited Pennywell Farm, a tourist attraction in South Devon. His pure nature was one of sensitivity, kindness and abhorrence of anything he didn't think was right. So, I believed that his decision to not eat meat was down to visiting the lovely cute little farm animals - a vegetarian on moral grounds.

I saw no reason to worry. I was perfectly aware of the need for Ollie to have balanced vegetarian meals, sufficient calcium, protein and minerals, especially as he was so young. Having once been a vegetarian for many years, I knew that vegetarianism, if practised appropriately, was a very healthy practice.

However, on reflection, had Ollie been an adolescent at the time of his conversion from carnivore to vegetarian, would I have been mindful of his motives and noticed any anorectic behaviour? To be honest, I think not. This act of morality was the start of a colossal collapse of my son's life and I welcomed it with open arms.

Weighing

Weighing is a healthy practice for some - but for those with an eating disorder, time on the bathroom scales can become a dangerous obsession.

It is common knowledge that a person's weight fluctuates throughout the day. There are a number of reasons for this, e.g. intake of fluid and food, and even the amount of urine held in the bladder - all of which are very natural processes and nothing to be concerned about. But someone with an eating disorder may not be as rational about the reasons for the weight changes. This lack of rationality could prove to be particularly distressing.

Weight fluctuation is an extremely disturbing matter for an anorexic to address, particularly if they weigh themselves. Initially, there is the fear and apprehension of weight gain. Once knowing the weight, there is the matter of trying to deal with thoughts of reducing intake further in an effort to weigh even less, which itself raises further anxiety and self-contempt.

When Ollie was discharged from the young person's psychiatric unit, a care plan was implemented stipulating who was going to be responsible for monitoring Ollie's vital statistics, which included a weekly weigh-in courtesy of his GP. Such weekly visits to the doctor were not without drama.

Ollie would begin to judder at the thought of his imminent visit. His hands would become hot and clammy. The colour would drain from him as he quivered nervously - almost as if he was going to pass out. Of course, the main factor driving his terror was the fear of uncovering his weight.

Being afraid of discovering his weight, or rather not wanting to hear how much weight he 'thought' he had gained throughout the week, Ollie tried a number of methods to avoid being confronted with the dreaded numbers. Furthermore, the frequent weigh-ins also revealed a conniving side to Ollie.

As time drew near for our jaunt to the doctors for the monitoring, Ollie would sometimes decide to change his clothes for the visit. Nothing wrong with wanting to look more presentable of course. However, it was not uncommon for him to change from light-weighted casual tracksuit bottoms into his heavily pocketed, chain-adorned pinstripe trousers, a number of layers on top and a host of studded wristbands.

Fortunately, I became aware of his underhand tactics, eventually took control of the game Ollie was playing and halted his attempts to manipulate the reading. It was an ingenious plot whilst he could get away with it - temporarily bumping up his natural weight for the monitoring session by wearing ludicrously heavy items. But what was even more crafty was that he sometimes hid items in his pockets for his extra benefit!

He would cooperate admirably with the exercises and other evidence related activities but, when it was time to monitor his weight, a different Ollie emerged in the consulting room.

The initial bravado waned and an anxious young man materialised. He employed a suite of strategies to help him cope with the unnerving situations such as mounting the scales backwards so that only the health professional could note the figures. Furthermore, he always reminded the health professional not to mention the findings out loud.

The fear of having his weight revealed to others has not waned throughout his journey to recovery. However, the way in which he managed this event for his own knowledge has - but not without shocking me in the process. Over time I discovered a series of receipts from the self-weigh facilities available in a high street store. But I think the most shocking discovery was the set of bathroom scales that Ollie had smuggled into his bedroom. Ollie's secret weighing practice could very easily have contributed to his mood swings and anxiety.

It is recommended that those recovering from anorexia should not weigh themselves more than once a week as it is a counterproductive practice. Indeed, it could be argued that self weighing is not necessary at all because of the close monitoring of the health professionals.

Yellowish skin

Anorexia has a devastating impact on all of the body's systems. The liver is one of the internal organs which can provide visible evidence of such an impact essentially through skin discolouration. The palms of the hands and soles of the feet turn sallow and wan. This is a condition called hypercarotinemia.[32]

In the case of hypercarotinemia, a non-toxic, temporary condition generally aligned to the excessive eating of foods containing carotene, e.g. carrots and papayas, the liver has problems converting carotenoids into Vitamin A (which is the vitamin important for growth and development, reproduction, immunity and many other functions). Consequently, any carotenoids not processed are deposited in the skin - hence the yellow tinge.

Even now, years after Ollie's admittance to hospital, I still have the vivid image of him and his emaciated yellow body on the hospital bed - and I continue to feel incredibly upset and traumatised.

8. MOVING FORWARD, LEARNING FROM MISTAKES

"With a heavy head and heart, a darkness shrouded me -

a darkness that was to last for years."

When Ollie was discharged from the young person's psychiatric unit due to his stay being 'detrimental to his recovery' - as was written on his care plan approach - the need to <u>fully</u> understand the intricacies of the enemy, anorexia, became an important focus of my life. I had been blindly thrust into the role of twenty-four seven carer and simultaneously stripped of my parenting role. To be able to effectively tend to my son's needs I needed to be suitably equipped with the knowledge base and appropriate skills.

As with any unit going into battle, the best way to fight the enemy is to be armed with information about it. In the early days of my son's diagnosis I responded to the rather poignant situation by embroiling myself in study. I wanted to learn as much as possible about anorexia - and I did. I commenced my battle strategy by scouring the internet - believe me there are a multitude of websites around, although not all of them are appropriate reading. However, one of the most informative and useful websites pertinent to our situation was the Men Get Eating Disorders Too website http://mengetedstoo.co.uk.

Men Get Eating Disorders Too is a UK charity founded by Sam Thomas, himself a recovered bulimia sufferer, who through his own experiences realised the need for a male specific resource. Ollie received a tremendous amount of support from Sam, and for that I will be forever grateful.

Unfortunately, support for me in my newly acquired role was virtually non-existent - I couldn't even obtain a carer's assessment. Information for carers of people battling an eating disorder was very patchy, especially in the South West of England. It was quite an exasperating time.

Nonetheless, as a social activist and not one to sit back and allow social injustice and unfairness to continue without challenge, I decided I had to do something about the lack of available support and information to me and others finding themselves in a similar situation.

I spent hours reflecting on my experiences around Ollie and anorexia. Yes, I was appalled at the varied level of care during his stay in the young person's psychiatric unit...and the negative effect it had on him. Furthermore, I felt incensed at the shortage of appropriate information and resources. So, I established No to Eating Disorders (NotED) http://www.noteduk.com, an information, awareness and support group for parents and carers of eating disordered children.

I found out relatively quickly, and not without tears, that communicating with an eating disordered person was not a simple process. People with eating disorders may misinterpret your words, or rather the eating disorder may twist them, particularly when you are trying to express concern. I had to rapidly reflect upon my abandoned knowledge and experiences as a health and social care lecturer in the hope that I held some useful tools in reserve. Luckily, I did.

I started to pay due attention to the way I talked with Ollie and began using 'I' statements and open questions. 'I' statements are excellent because they enable you to state calmly and clearly what you are thinking and feeling, and why. Leaving very little room for misunderstanding, the risk of confrontation and arguments is drastically reduced - and open questions not only pass control of the conversation over to the respondent but they also facilitate honesty and foster respect between the individuals.

Such questioning also encourages a safe, non-threatening environment. I often wonder had I used the open questioning technique with Ollie before he received a diagnosis whether some of his teenage years might have been spent differently.

It was usual for Ollie to spend Saturdays out with his friends. He would return home about 9pm, plonk himself in front of the television and that would be it for the night. As he settled, I would ask him the concerned and interested parent questions, such as "Did you have a nice time?" and "Where did you go?" He would casually answer, mentioning in not too great a detail, some of the things that he and his friends had been up to, including how they had purchased and scoffed packs of doughnuts or eaten a McDonald's meal - but he hadn't. Consequently, when I followed up such information by asking him if he had eaten, the reply was always a sharp, resounding yes - no further discussion required.

Regrettably, I have since uncovered a sinister account of the Saturday mealtimes out. But first of all, I have to stress that Ollie hadn't lied to me, it is more a case of misleading me.

Ollie has revealed that although he had eaten, his consumption was sometimes no more than one chocolate Malteser! I feel sure that proficiency in open questioning could well have seriously halted some of the restrictive eating taking place or, at the very least, I could have worked harder on encouraging him to eat when he returned home.

Conversations were indeed demanding at times. Ollie would occasionally become rude, impolite or aggressive - quite out of character behaviour which, rightly or wrongly, I firmly placed at the door of the anorexia. Consequently any reproaches addressing such behaviour had to be put on hold until a more appropriate opportunity to discuss the events arose. I learnt very quickly to prepare myself for a brief talk rather than a full blown conversation.

Mealtimes were exceptionally daunting occasions - for Ollie and for me. As anorexia isn't a fan of food, Ollie's anxiety levels rocketed and the tension in the house equalled it. Ollie knew he had to face his fear on the plate, but my fear was twofold - the unpredictability of Ollie's reactions to the food on his plate and any dinner table discussions.

Speaking from experience, and the desire to protect people from similar distressing encounters, please steer discussions away from food related topics, including portion sizes, calorie content of food stuffs and such like...and this includes any references to food on your own plate. You do not want to initiate 'intake comparisons' and feelings of guilt.

As with all learning curves, I made so many mistakes. When Ollie was struggling with the meal in front of him I used to say things like, "Try a little bit more for me." just to get an extra, life-preserving, morsel in his mouth. But this gentle cajoling was wrong. I was using Ollie's love and affection for me as a tool for blackmail. My pathetic attempts at encouraging him to eat more simply added pressure to an already pressurised situation.

Another one of my mistakes was praising him for eating well. I thought I was offering words of encouragement and support for future endeavours, but I was making Ollie feel guilty for what he had eaten. But it wasn't only Ollie's guilt at eating that I had to contend with - I had to deal with my own.

As previously mentioned, eating disorders are coping strategies which develop over time as a consequence of one, or a combination of emotional, psychological, social, inter-personal or biological factors. No guilt or blame should be attached to any one person or situation - but that is easier said than done. I can't adequately express the guilt I felt for Ollie's suffering.

The more I learnt and understood about anorexia, the more pain and guilt I felt. I repeatedly beat myself up for not noticing the obvious tell-tale signs. With a heavy head and heart, a darkness shrouded me - a darkness that was to last for years.

I became a master at hiding my turmoil - but in the end had to succumb to the need for professional help. It took a considerable amount of therapy and medication before I could begin to put the feelings of guilt and blame aside.

There were times when I just wanted to put my arms around Ollie, squeeze him tight and absorb all of his terrible pain and suffering. Sadly, there was a significant obstacle in the way - his poor body image. The ruthless and negative way in which he regarded his body resulted in him not only shying away from any personal approaches, but also increased his feeling of unworthiness for any show of affection.

I recall how Ollie used to cringe when I, or anyone else for that matter, wanted to show signs of affection. He would hunch his shoulders and bring his whole being together, making himself as small and insignificant as possible. He would lower his head deep into his chest and, with eyes full of dread, plead 'No'. I know that this negative reaction to affection is not uncommon.

Indeed, many parents have commented on the hurt they experienced when their eating disordered child rejected their affectionate approaches - but likewise on their joy and elation when receiving the all important first unsolicited hug!

Each time Ollie rejected my show of affection, I felt as if my heart had been ripped out, leaving a gaping chasm within my chest. It never got any easier. Obviously I was hurt, but deep down I knew that there were reasons for his actions. Fortunately, one thing that the anorexia hadn't taken away from us was our ability to, albeit occasionally, talk openly about matters.

Ollie divulged his hatred of his body; how he hated touching his own body because of the fat, rolls and rolls of fat, which disgusted him. Although I felt shocked by the way he felt, I consoled him the only way I knew how - by expressing how much I loved him, despite the difficult times we were experiencing.

I accept this may not have been easy for Ollie to hear because of his self-adorned unworthiness. However, sometimes I needed a hug to help me through the day and I mentioned that. He bashfully admitted that occasionally he needed a hug too! Dispensing with the beauty of spontaneity we agreed that should ever either one of us want a hug, we just needed to ask.

A vast amount of the time I felt completely helpless. I struggled incessantly with not being able to fix my broken son. But I was not his therapist. I was not the one to mend his body and mind. My role was to remain the provider of endless love and support.

The website of Beat, the UK's leading eating disorder charity, mentioned that everyone who has recovered from an eating disorder has said how important the unconditional love received from their family and friends was throughout their journey.[33]

Of course, unconditional love might sound like a given in respect of a parent's love for their child, but eating disorders create so much distress, disharmony and frustration that the challenging times faced are nothing like anything before experienced - tempers, feelings and situations could become strained, abundantly so.

Unconditional love is exactly as it states - love without conditions. No strings attached. No demands. No expectations - just love, respect and acceptance for being the person they are - regardless.

9. A NEW HOPE

"Recovery offered an opportunity to live life as one really should, driving one's own destiny and not being the back seat passenger."

Recovery from an eating disorder is possible. However, the process is more complicated than simply taking medication - or no longer needing medication. It requires support with the medical, psychological, emotional and behavioural transformations (changes which may be quite scary) that are going to occur.

As mentioned in a previous chapter, I herald the day my son was diagnosed with anorexia. In my eyes, that was the day my son started the road to recovery. A diagnosis meant access to appropriate treatments, therapies and regular monitoring. It was also the beginning of a new era of understanding among family and friends that Ollie was indeed seriously ill. Unfortunately, Ollie didn't respond favourably to the resulting attention from professionals. Nonetheless, he endured whatever the professionals dictated - but it wasn't until he really wanted to recover, it wasn't until he had acquired a particular mindset, that his recovery journey commenced.

Narratives musing over recovery from eating disorders discuss salient personal turning points for the start of the recovery journey. Events can be as instantaneous as a reflection or the enduring work of an exemplary, supportive health professional. Ollie's turning point was when he turned eighteen. Becoming eighteen didn't only mark his transition into adulthood, it was a light bulb moment that changed his whole outlook.

This special birthday delivered a great present for all of us - optimism. He transformed into an exceptionally upbeat young man. We had discussions centring on when, not if, he recovered. Talk about a future eradicated his past comments about wanting to die.

His new-found sanguinity revealed his desire to see the end of anorexia. It was music to my ears, and not because I was yearning to stop my persistent worrying about him - to be honest, as parents do we ever stop worrying? Neither was it to see the end of his occasionally disturbing obsessions with food. It was because Ollie would be able to sculpt a new life, free from all of the psychological constraints and severe physical consequences that the anorexia had imposed on him.

Ollie had spent years living an illusion. Through his restrictive eating behaviour he thought he was in control of his life, but he was wrong - anorexia was controlling him. Recovery offered an opportunity to live life as one really should, driving one's own destiny and not being the back seat passenger. Despite his positive disposition, the anorexia wasn't going to suddenly dissipate. Recovery is dependent upon a number of factors, all pertinent to the individual.

A person's recovery journey is as individual as the person is unique. However, the actual recovery process can be narrowed down into a number of stages of change. At this point I believe it is germane to mention the matter of relapse.

There are different trains of thought regarding the subject of relapse. Relapse is widely discussed in context of recovery. Some consider relapse an important part of the recovery process which, although terribly disheartening and disempowering, can be viewed as important elements to gaining strength and building skills to cope with the challenges of the daunting process.

Others advocate relapse prevention as critical to recovery and therefore do not include it as part of the recovery cycle. With this in mind I will briefly introduce the general five stages of change in recovery.

The first stage of recovery is pre-contemplation. Here the person is unable to accept, or quite profusely denies, that their behaviour is problematic (for example, purging via excessive exercising). Consequently, they demonstrate no intention to change.

Contemplation, the second stage, is where the person may start to seriously consider changing their behaviours, but display a hesitancy in doing anything about it - which could provoke moments of pure frustration and confusion. The preparation stage can be very stressful and full of anxiety - for the eating disordered person and those supporting. Here the preparations to make those all important necessary changes to behaviour are made.

The action stage of recovery is where the eating disordered person will challenge their unhealthy behaviour by implementing the plans from the preparation stage. This stage is particularly difficult and it is vital that the support network is strong, determined and encouraging. Relapses are commonplace in this stage as the person is confronting fears and experimenting with new behaviours whilst working on discarding the old unhealthy ones.

Once the person has managed to sustain their new behaviour and healthier thinking processes for a number of months, they will enter into the maintenance stage, where the newly-acquired self-caring skills and knowledge are also used. Again, it is possible for the person to experience relapses.

Absorbing the facets of recovery, I consequently prepared myself for a long, arduous roller coaster ride of emotions. Ollie had been hiding under a blanket of iniquitous comforts of fear, anxiety, mistrust and isolation for many years. Through recovery, his safety blanket was going to lose its threads. His non-idealistic, ritualistic world would soon be exposed to the real world - and he was going to feel threatened and afraid.

I had to ready myself for the perceived turbulent times ahead - the shifts in moods and angry words. But, I also had to prime Ollie to harness any motivation and positivity, and encourage him to keep it in store for the demoralising days. I appreciate that it was not my recovery. Nonetheless, I understood how important it was for me to believe in Ollie's recovery, to support him through the rough and smooth of the process, particularly through the relapses.

Of course, I was not the only person providing support to my son at this time. A whole host of health professionals were concerned with his journey. The GP provided relief from anorexia's various sidekicks via prescription medication. This proved very problematic as, in the beginning, Ollie refused to take antidepressants. He feared the possible side effects, or rather one - that of weight gain.

Ollie attended numerous therapies, not only for anorexia but also body dysmorphia. Initially, Ollie attended Cognitive Behavioural Therapy (CBT). This type of therapy, which has three phases, is considered a significant part of the recovery process because of its attention to the required skills and education to eventually heal oneself of the eating disorder.

However, the complexities of Ollie's individuality advocated a different therapy, Dialectical Behavioural Therapy (DBT), which included the learning of four sets of skills - mindfulness, interpersonal effectiveness, emotion regulation and distress tolerance. For those not fully au fait with mindfulness, mindfulness is a simple ancient Buddhist concept which encourages individuals to seek a new way of not only interacting with their world but accepting it. Through exercises and skills building, individuals become more aware of their feelings and thoughts in the moment.

The interpersonal effectiveness feature of DBT however, focuses on an individual's assertiveness. Here skills around one's objective effectiveness (obtaining what the individual wants effectively) are explored as are skills designed to maintain and improve relationships. A further element of interpersonal effectiveness is the honing of skills around self respect.

Emotional regulation provides insight into how emotions work and explores the skills required to manage them. Whereas, Distress Tolerance looks at the development of skills to assist with coping and surviving a crisis - very personal facets of any individual!

I truly appreciate how hard and arduously the therapists worked with Ollie. I am grateful to them for facilitating the development of his skills base. Indeed even today, Ollie calls upon some of the learned skills. Mindfulness was a particularly useful tool for Ollie, and I must admit that I found the practice invaluable for my own journey out of the black mire.

Furthermore, I feel I must also pay credit to the dietician for her role in Ollie's journey. As well as assisting with the ditching of some rather distorted views of food, she helped him abandon some of his invented dietary rules. But, more importantly to me, she provided him with accurate nutritional information, in part through the references to academic research, which enabled Ollie to construct an objective correlation of nutrition and the body.

I recall his passionate retelling of the 1945 year-long Minnesota Starvation Experiment, led by Dr. Ancel Keys, on the impact of malnutrition upon the body. Although Ollie had lived through starvation and was continuing to deal with the negative effects, this research really intrigued him.[34]

Briefly, the Minnesota Starvation Experiment used the services of thirty-six healthy, young, conscientious objectors to the Second World War. The study comprised of three phases. The first phase normalised intake at 3200 calories a day for a period of three months. The second phase introduced a reduced daily consumption of 1570 calories for six months (starvation stage), with the final phase being rehabilitation. This may seem strange, but I found Ollie's interest in this study a further indicator of the, albeit slow, progress he was making.

Occasionally Ollie's journey was a very troublesome time for me. Alongside the continued anxiety attacks, moodiness, aches and pains, Ollie found solace in an extremely negative coping strategy - alcohol. He took to drinking rather frequently and heavily - well, the calories consumed through alcohol meant (to him) he didn't have to eat. But it wasn't only Ollie's behaviour that worried me, so too did the reactions of family and friends to his obvious signs of recovery - in particular, his weight gain.

People were extremely zealous with their praises and congratulatory comments regarding Ollie's fresh, healthy appearance. I would have openly welcomed their observations had my son been recovering from flu. However, I have to admit to feeling rather uncomfortable and sometimes cringing, when such instances arose.

Distorted thoughts, particularly around body image, do not automatically disappear once recovery has started. In recovery, as when in the grip of anorexia, any comments on appearance or weight can be misconstrued as 'looking fat' (something the anorexic deeply fears) and thereby trigger the adverse eating-disordered thoughts and practices.

There is a great deal of learning required by the person in recovery to recognise that the black and white thinking is unhealthy - and a great deal of skill in making such thoughts invalid to their lives.

It is important to state that, just because someone appears to have a healthy weight by no way does it mean that the turmoil of the eating disorder is over. Gaining weight is only one facet of the recovery process for someone with an eating disorder. Issues around the emotional and psychological circumstance of the individual also need to be addressed - such issues may require months or even years of specialised attention.

Therefore despite people's best intentions, any comments to, or about my son, had a tendency to not only upset him but also disrupt, quite devastatingly, the course of his recovery. I must say that we had some very hairy moments trying to manage the aftermath of well-intended acclaim...and other triggers.

Despite the occasional blips, Ollie continued on the rather jagged path of recovery whilst I remained forever vigilant of him stumbling into the mire of unwholesome practices again. But not all of my son's journey was draining - some instances were positively uplifting.

One such moment, and I believe quite a significant gauge to test the process of his recovery, was when he thrust upon me his desire to move away from his home city. Undeniably, I was aghast at the revelation - but none more so than when he declared he wanted to move to London, nearly two hundred miles away.

Of course, leaving Plymouth would provide a fantastic opportunity for a truly independent life - after all, independence is a key feature to aid recovery! It would be a fresh start for him. He could form a new identity away from the things and places he associated with anorexia, including the people that previously tagged him with the now unwanted label of anorexic. But, my heart sank as I foresaw some serious implications for his recovery with this intended move.

My knowledge of mental health services in London was zilch, let alone the eating disorder services. I very much doubted whether Ollie knew any different. I questioned whether he would even attempt to engage with the much-needed services anyway.

In addition, there was the issue of the practicalities of independent living in a bustling, expensive, cosmopolitan city - accommodation, travel, entertainment and leisure, food.

Regardless of the lack of enthusiasm I had for Ollie's proposed move to the capital, he had finally started to visualise a future for himself - and it was one free of the eating disorder. And, despite my internal protestations, I thoroughly accepted that Ollie needed to build a new life for himself - as did I, for the past few years had been extremely demanding, exasperating and daunting for both of us. So, as any loving and caring mother would, I gave Ollie's idea considerable thought. Months later he moved to Exeter, a mere forty-seven miles away. A superb compromise! Ollie would be distanced enough to be liberated from worried eyes and I was content in the knowledge that should negative thinking and irrationality begin once again to play with his mind, I was less than an hour's journey away should I ever be needed.

Finally, after enduring extensive conflict with poor health, pain, distress and despair, my youngest child felt strong enough to commandeer his own life. I felt blessed and victorious. Although my war with Ollie's anorexia was not over, my triumph was for Ollie. His latest mindset indicated a powerful determination for change. His skirmishes with the vicious eating disorder were nearing an end.

Anorexia had imposed a miserable existence upon me - in fact, its venom affected everyone in my family. However, the harsh experiences only served to diminish my eternal flame of belief in a better future - one of hope - not douse it. Admittedly, there were times when forlorn hope was waiting to overwhelm me, particularly when Ollie lay immobile in a hospital bed attached to ECG sensors.

Anorexia may have robbed me of watching my youngest son enjoy his teenage years without pain and suffering. Anorexia may have incarcerated my son with its vicious falsehoods and vile tricks. Furthermore, anorexia may have stripped him of his happy childhood memories, so much so that he cannot recollect any feelings or emotions whilst glancing through the family photographs.

Ollie's resurgence from the dark mire of anorexia rekindled my inner flame, so much so that my body tingled with exhilarating hope. As Archbishop Desmond Tutu, social rights activist and Nobel Peace Prize winner once said, "Hope is being able to see that there is light despite all of the darkness." - and he was right.

But my hope not only helped me see through the darkest of times, it helped me build an armoury with weapons of fortitude, strength and sanguinity, all stored in preparation for life's future battles and wars.

REFERENCES

1. Bryant-Waugh, R. & Lask, B. (2004) Eating Disorders. A Parents' Guide. East Sussex: Brunner-Routledge

2. Sato, T. & McCann, D. (2007) "Sociotropy–autonomy and interpersonal problems", *Depression and Anxiety* (Wiley-LISS) **24** (3): 153–162, doi:10.1002/da.20230, retrieved 9 April 2014

3. University of Windsor, Scholarship at UWindsor, Electronic Theses and Dissertations. 1-1-1998, Relations of autonomy and sociotropy to eating disturbances in female university students and women with eating disorders. Karen Joan. Narduzzi University of Windsor

4. Middleton, K. (2007) Eating Disorders. The Path To Recovery. Oxford: Lion Hudson plc.

5. Nasser, M., Katzman, M., & Gordon, R. (2001). Eating disorders and cultures in transition. London: Brunner-Routledge

6. Kayrooz, C. (2001) A systemic treatment of bulimia nervosa. Women in transition. London: Jessica Kingsley Publishers

7. Bell, R.M. (1987) Holy Anorexia. University of Chicago Press: Chicago

8. Buser, J.K. & Woodford, M.S. (2010) Eating Disorders/Spiritual Beliefs. Professional Counseling Digest. American Counseling Association

URL: https://www.counseling.org/docs/default-source/library-archives/professional-counselor-digest/acapcd-35.pdf?sfvrsn=4

9. Szmukler, G.I., et.al. (1986) Anorexia Nervosa and Bulimic Disorder. Current Perspectives. Pergamon Press Ltd. Oxford

10. American Psychiatric Association. (2013). Diagnostic and statistical manual of mental disorders (5th ed.).

11. Keating, C. et al. (2012) Reward processing in anorexia nervosa. Neuropsychologia 50 (2012) 567–575

URL:http://www.srossell.com/Publications/51%20keating%20anorexia%20neuropsychologia%202012.pdf

12. Best-Boss, A. (2012) The Everything Parent's Guide to Eating Disorders. USA: F+W Media

13. http://alzonline.phhp.ufl.edu/en/reading/Anosognosia.pdf

14.http://www.rcpsych.ac.uk/healthadvice/problemsdisorders/bipolardisorder.aspx

15. Craggs-Hinton, C. (2006) Coping with Eating Disorders and Body Image. London: Sheldon Press

16. http://www.borderline-personality-disorder.com/co-occuring-disorders/eating-disorders/

17. http://psychcentral.com/disorders/dependent-personality-disorder-symptoms/

18. Boachie, A. & Jasper, K. (2011) A Parent's Guide to Defeating Eating Disorders. London: Jessica Kingsley Publishers

19. https://www.psychologytoday.com/conditions/histrionic-

personality-disorder

20. Tompkins, M.A. (2012). OCD: A Guide for the Newly Diagnosed. Oakland: New Harbinger

21. http://psychcentral.com/news/2010/10/10/eating-disorders-linked-to-self-harm/19404.html

22. Herrin, M. & Matsumoto, N. (2002) The Parent's Guide to Childhood Eating Disorders New York:Henry Holt & Co.

23. http://www.livestrong.com/article/502638-sorbitol-and-bloating-from-gas/

24. http://www.livestrong.com/article/522867-eating-disorders-gum-chewing/

25. http://www.remudaranch.com/

26.http://www.youngminds.org.uk/for_parents/whats_worrying_you_about_your_child/self-esteem/about_self-esteem

27. http://umm.edu/health/medical/reports/articles/eating-disorders

28. http://healthyeating.sfgate.com/ghrelin-levels-rise-leptin-levels-fall-7536.html

29. Byatnal, K. (2012) Extreme Conditions - How The Brain Fights Starvation. URL:http://www.luxperci.com/extreme-conditions-how-the-brain-fights-starvation

30. Challem, J. (2006) The Food-Mood Connection URL:https://experiencelife.com/article/the-food-mood-connection/

31. Quick, V. & Byrd-Bredbenner, C. (2013) Vegetarians and Vegans: Are They at Increased Risk for Disordered Eating and Poor Psychological Well-Being? Journal of the Academy of Nutrition and Dietetics, Vol. 113, Issue 9, Supplement

32. Smoller, B. R. & Rongioletti, F. (2010) Clinical and Pathological Aspects of Skin Diseases in Endocrine, Metabolic, Nutritional and Deposition Disease. New York: Springer

33. http://www.b-eat.co.uk/about-eating-disorders/worried-about-someone

34. http://www.apa.org/monitor/2013/10/hunger.aspx

ABOUT THE AUTHOR

Debbie Roche, mother of three, is a former health and social care lecturer. Distressing experiences encouraged her to move into the mental health arena where she sits on various strategic boards.

Utilising her lived experiences and theoretical knowledge of anorexia, Debbie founded No to Eating Disorders (NotED), an eating disorder awareness and support group. http://www.noteduk.com

An accredited Mental Health First Aid trainer, Debbie also delivers a diverse range of mental health related awareness courses.

Although Debbie has seen some of her poetry in print, this is her first book.

Originally from Sheffield, Debbie now lives in Plymouth.